The Dwindling

A DAUGHTER'S CAREGIVING JOURNEY TO
THE EDGE OF LIFE

JANET DUNNETT

Journeys Press

Published by Journeys Press

Journeys Press
543 Rowan Drive,
Qualicum Beach,
British Columbia
Canada
V9K 1K1
www.journeyspress.ca

Library and Archives Canada Cataloguing in Publication

Dunnett, Janet, author
The dwindling : a daughter's caregiving journey to the edge of life
/ Janet Dunnett.

ISBN 978-0-9958644-1-2 (softcover)

1. Dunnett, Janet--Family. 2. Daughters--Family relationships--
Canada. 3. Twins--Family relationships--Canada. 4. Adult children of
aging parents--Canada--Biography. 5. Aging parents--Care--Canada.

I. Title.

HQ1064.C3D86 2017   306.874092   C2017-900253-8

Cover design: Fiona Dunnett at www.fionadunnett.com
Typeset in *Berling* at SpicaBookDesign

Printed in Canada

To Judi
We are the twin team

Note to Readers

Though the dialogue in this narrative is a reconstruction of my memory of the kinds of things people said and how they said them, each chapter begins with my mother's actual words.

I have changed names and places except for my family and the care locations where this story happened.

Goliath represents all large health care bureaucracies challenged to get it right when delivering quality care at the edge of life.

Special Thanks

I owe a debt of gratitude to all my sources of strength as I lived the dwindling time and then wrote about it afterwards.

First and foremost, I thank my twin sister, Judi, my womb mate. Through it all and beyond we are the twin team.

My husband Ed was patient and quietly supportive through the dwindling years when I spent more time in Calgary than on the Coast with him. Then, as I needed to write the story on my own, he held back giving advice and accepted my decision not to share the drafts. Thank you for standing by.

My children are a source of my strength. My son Jamie stepped in when I needed his hands-on help through the dwindling time. His eyes-wide-open view of the Parent Project guided the twin team. But it was Fiona, my daughter, who never failed to ask, "But how are YOU doing, Mom?" and for that tenderness and care for the caregiver, I am forever grateful. Her illustration on my cover captures the feeling of the time in a way no other person in the world could.

I acknowledge that all my siblings and family did their very best to be there for Fred and Betty and for the twin team, too. If there were times when we did not see eye to eye, there were never times when we were not heart to heart.

In learning how to write this narrative, I turned to friends to read earlier versions. They gave good advice. There was Judi, but also Carol Merchasin, Janet Howey and Cherie Rae Wright. I've had the special attention and editing skill of Kristin Masters, and the support of Iryna Spica in book design. I thank them all for their friendship as well as their love of ideas well captured and presented. My sister Nancy Strider shared some of her favourite photographs to help me convey the tenderness that was part of the dwindling time.

The vast machine called Alberta Health Services is full of skilled and sensitive people. Though I often felt powerless lobbing my advocacy pebbles at this Goliath, I am also grateful that it was there. I know that without this giant doing its best, my parents might have missed what quality of life they had in the dwindling time.

Prologue

"It is what it is."

I know I was not the first grey-haired child in history to hurtle into a crowded Emergency Room trailing behind a stretcher, fizzing in shame as everyone turned to look. But on a hot August night in 2008, with my mother banging the rails of her stretcher and screaming that I was killing her, I felt all alone.

Later that night, a chubby intern with thick glasses said not to worry. Mom probably had an infection. Perhaps her metabolism had become sluggish, so the right dose last week of one or another of her many pills was an overdose now. He shrugged. "It's very common. Meds get tricky with old girls like your mother." He scribbled something on his clipboard. Without another word, he jabbed a needle into Mom's upper arm as she screamed in shock. "This will calm her down." My relief was seasoned with a dash of irritation. Why did doctors tell daughters not to worry when they brought their hallucinating parents to Emergency in the middle of the night, as if more intelligent caregivers would not be so quick to overreact? And why didn't they tell us what new medication they were pumping into our loved ones on top of everything else already inside them? And what was this bit about calling an octogenarian an old girl? I knew by this stage of the caregiver game that tongue-biting worked better than tongue-lashing. But it all got me thinking.

Within days of that awful night, my mother was back to her sweet self, telling me what a good daughter I was and how much she appreciated having me around. I breathed easier, but I couldn't shake a dawning insight. If my trauma was garden-variety, then there must be a tribe of us out there, unpaid family caregivers, probably feeling belittled, confused and isolated by conditions just like I was in. "Nothing to worry about" was probably twisting all our lives in knots.

I was right on. There are a lot of us. Statistics Canada says that an estimated 28% of my fellow citizens over the age of 15 are currently looking after family members or friends with long-term health conditions, disability or aging needs, and 39% of those caregivers are tending their parents. That's about the same as our American neighbours. A silver tsunami is on its way, with we baby boomers hitting the age of 65 at a rate of 1,000 a day in Canada. People over 85 are the fastest-growing segment of the American population. The numbers are all there. It is not, as the doctor said, "Nothing to worry about."

The tribe of family caregivers has far more women members than men, for now at least. Is there some tag on a gene for caregiving that is epigenetically slower to switch on in men? Perhaps it is simply the way we are socialized as little girls. Whatever our sex, though, it is a safe bet that most of us didn't see the job coming, or wanted it when it did. Most important, few of us had any training in the complex tasks involved to take it on, let alone thrive.

Is there anything special about this caregiving daughterhood? I think we understand each other. Though most of us are far too busy in our personal cocoons of calamity to share our stories, we suspect in our guts that what scientists say is fact. In crisis, we women tend and befriend, while men are hardwired to shake their fists at the threat, or else make a run for it. That makes us willing caregivers. We women also admit more readily to our feelings of fear, fury or futility, while men seem more often to be trapped in bravado. I see the daughterhood everywhere.

In a crowded elevator last year, I nodded at a wrinkled baby boomer, while all the men stared straight ahead. I observed her holding up her even more shriveled parent while studying her wristwatch and grimacing, and felt a wave of empathy toward her. "Going to an appointment with your mother?" I asked.

"Yes, how did you know?" she answered, looking shocked.

"I just do," I replied.

Yup, I thought. That's the daughterhood effect.

In a grocery store, I chatted with the lady ahead of me in the line pushing an economy-sized package of adult diapers through the till and looking sheepish, like I used to as a teenager buying Tampax. She admitted the diapers were for her mother and told me how her mom wasn't making it to the bathroom in time, so there were "accidents." She blushed. I said my mother had the same problem. "It's called functional incontinence." She nodded and I added, "It's common in elderly women." She was impressed, she said, at what I knew, and I felt a flush of pride. It was true. I love Dr. Google and getting lost following all the links from one set of facts to others. I'm sure I know more about the ins and outs of advanced aging than most non-medical types with less curiosity. The woman and I riffed back and forth about the whole situation being stinky, and then we laughed. The cashier moved the bundle along and said her mother wore diapers, too, extra absorbent. She told us where she bought them cheaper. Right on! I thought with a smile, there it is again. The daughterhood effect.

In that midnight dash with Mom's delirium, I noticed that many of the plastic chairs in the outback of the emergency room were occupied by keening ancients, with drawn-faced women patting their gnarled hands. I heard one whisper, "Don't worry, Mom, I think you are next," and knew that couldn't be true. No old person still conscious could have a problem bigger in that triage world than the young men dripping blood from their stab wounds or the suits clutching their chests as they arrived. I knew frail old people and their daughters regularly lingered for hours at the back of the queue. Was that fair? I wondered. Now the paramedics wheeled my mother right past this couple and through the doors to be checked in. Judi and I knew from frequent experience never to take Mom or Dad to Emergency any other way than by ambulance. Stretchers got a head start in the race to care. Should I have given the daughter that hint for her inevitable next time? I wondered, too, why she wasn't more assertive with the triage nurse. Didn't she know about squeaky wheels? Part of me wanted to stop, but Mom was hollering about me putting poison in the water, so I followed her stretcher out of the public eye. I guess someone has to go last, I thought. Still, I felt the daughterhood effect.

Daughters or not, we family caregivers are lacerated by our grip on a two-edged sword. On one side are statistics that show life is lasting longer. An array of medical marvels and slick systems now fend off sudden death, or at least make sure that we stagger on with a host of non-terminal conditions. Our world is safer, too, with our seat belts and smoke alarms and expiry dates on the yogurt. Quick ends from strokes or heart attacks, or demises from failing organs, diseases or infections are rarer, at least in Western societies. What was fatal for my grandmother is a pesky chronic condition now. But Nature always wins. That's the other side of the bloody blade. Life in the last years is a messy stew of maladies that pile on, one after another, and can't be cured. They all cause suffering. Most adults of advanced age struggle with their list of co-morbidities until one little something becomes the big one, and they are suddenly gone, leaving bewildered care-givers to say, "She was doing so well until..." We agree that slow death is no life for a human, but as a society we're flum-moxed about what to do as the social order reshapes itself from mostly youthful to mostly old.

We boomers are masters of denial. We'll be lucky and have a quick stroke or some terminal diagnosis that carries us off without a long goodbye. Better yet, we'll get hit by lightning on the golf course. We are magical thinkers, too, assuming every problem has a solution, and why not? Since we first squalled our way into the world, our generation has forced all the changes we needed to fit our good life and evolving world views. There was birth control, divorce, abor-tion, pensions, and recently same-sex marriage, and in Canada there are new laws that let doctors help some of us check out when we've had enough of life and not risk jail time.

Those of us who are or have been family caregivers know that advocacy is needed to change anything. But we are too tired after it is over or too busy getting on with our lives to consider ourselves as part of that solution. In our inaction we still share one concern, though. "What will happen when my turn comes to dwindle?"

That's why I wrote this memoir. When my father faded and finally died in late December 2009 at the age of 92, and my mother followed a year later, aged 88 and far more infirm for far longer, I wanted to forget the whole thing at first. I had a bucket list I'd set aside for a decade. But forgetting wasn't as easy as wanting to. As I gained distance and no longer saw their dying selves in my mind's eye, but their vibrant selves before the dwindling, I realized that there were far more rewards in caregiving than I appreciated in the middle of the job. Even more wondrous, I saw how my tenderness toward them had expanded as they grew more vulnerable. Our family dance of being cared for and giving the care had changed me. Maybe my making a small difference in the world came from making a big difference to my parents.

Slow dying also opened reasons and ways to reconnect with my siblings. We re-learned about each other's lives and found a deeper version of intimacy than was ever possible as kids competing for parent resources or in our adult diaspora. I had doubted I could ever be closer to my identical twin sister Judi than I had always been. But I was wrong about that, too. We co-created the Parent Project. She was Daughter on Deck and I was Daughter at a Distance and we always had each other's back. We knew that our caregiving for Mom and Dad was the right thing for us to do. We were the twin team.

There will be many responses to my story of family caregiving.

"I'm sure not going to read someone else's sob story. I have my own."

"Gee whiz, that happened to me, too!"

"Aw, come on! That was not my experience!"

"Hmmm…I must give that a try."

"There's got to be a better way!"

Something has got to shift in the way our health systems approach care at the end of life. Whatever the reaction to this story, I hope it contributes to the power of shared experience that can make change happen.

There are risks. Others with bit parts in my story of Judi and me, Mom and Dad, might say I have got it all wrong. After all, Fred and Betty raised seven kids who each had a unique relationship with them. We each saw their dwindling time through our personal points of view. What we remember and what we forget is individual. But I have my truth.

A library of notebooks, and gigabytes of emails never trashed both jog and confirm my memory. The entries set out what happened when, and many take a stab at why. I didn't carry around a tape recorder so the dialogue is the gist of the story. Other than my siblings, I changed most names and places. It's all about privacy. The most significant name change is also the biggest actor in this narrative about life and gradual death. Alberta Health Services is an archetype of any health bureaucracy. I called it Goliath. It is huge, well-intentioned, but often with blind spots. We family caregivers, trifling Davids, have little more than our personal experience as ammunition in our advocacy slingshots. But, as in the Bible story, David gets his point across to Goliath in the end.

Calgary, Alberta, is the sprawling oil capital of Canada. Its rush hours and traffic snarls made the bouncing between Mom and Dad into a daily odyssey. Qualicum Beach is my idyllic home town on the edge of continental Canada in British Columbia. It faces the better-known city of Vancouver across 32 miles of ocean. My parents referred to my town as the Coast, so I do, too. Most Canadians think of my province, British Columbia, as Lotus Land, "a place inducing contentment," as Google puts it. That's sure how Mom and Dad saw it.

But I'm getting ahead of myself. My story of caring for Betty and Fred did not actually begin the night I didn't murder Mom. It started years before. As the calendar flipped from one millennium to the next, I spent three transformational days with my mother. That's where I begin.

Table of Contents

1

Three Days

"I told you not to fuss!"

Mom held out her coffee mug for a refill, leaving room for her cream-o and fake sugar. We looked out at the dawn and agreed that whatever weather this last day of 1999 would bring, tempting bright blue sky or gusts of blowing snow, we wouldn't budge. We sipped and snuggled at opposite ends of the sofa, tugging our one blanket back and forth between us and tucking pillows behind our backs just so, to watch the television. There was that nerve-scratching jingle again. It announced the very-big-deal global collaboration to bring the moment of the new millennium to our living rooms from around the world, in real time. Mom and I were excited about it. I was also worried. Would the moment of the Millennium bring on the Bug? Would its bite paralyze us all? In my job developing policy for the Canadian government, Y2K had ground me down for months. I didn't understand the details. In the Year 2000, computers would get confused, I was assured, and then shut down. It was something about code and the number 2. I'd brought all my files home for the Christmas holiday with Mom, "just in case." Finally, we would know. The first time zone to reach the New Year was deep in the Pacific, but Australia kicked off the broadcast. I clutched my mug as the ruddy Australian came on with his "G'day, Mates" and news that elevators still ran in Sydney, money machines still spit out cash, and the lights were on Down Under. Y2K was a hoax, he hinted. Mom gurgled with glee. "I told you not to fuss!" She reminded me that I worried too much about things that hadn't happened. Hadn't she said all along that Y2K was malarkey and we were all suckers to fall for it? I let her gloat.

Mom did live in the moment and generally didn't worry about what hadn't happened yet. Except for Christmas. Every year in barbecue season she would hint that she was getting edgy about being alone for the holidays. Every year my six siblings checked in on the one common issue of the time: Who would invite Mom? It was always me.

"You don't have to entertain me," Mom always insisted. But I did. Always, I was her acolyte for the week or two she overwhelmed our family agenda. I kept fresh coffee coming in the morning and switched to rum and Coke once the sun was over the yardarm, as she put it, noon on the dot. At night I brewed chamomile tea for her to sip as she soaked in her bath made fragrant with lavender oil, her favorite scent. I emptied her ashtray before it was full and, most of all, kept the fire burning. When she dozed on the sofa, I rushed to finish my family chores and get dinner ready. The holidays exhausted me but I cherished every one. We were lethargic this time, playing endless Scrabble and watching repeats of *Jeopardy* or more highbrow fare like *Masterpiece Theatre*. Mom's back and hips and neck were bothering her. Catering to her, caring for her, was my version of love.

The truth was, I wasn't sure what love actually looked like other than selfless service. I didn't have many models. Our parents had never been what we called mushy with each other or with us. Getting seven kids to functional adulthood was testament to a partnership that worked, though. That was love. Mom said Dad's family didn't know about hugging so his emotional stiffness was an inherited trait. Mom was the really distant parent, though, at least in my preschooler memory. She was happy when her nose was in a book or a pen was in her inky right hand, scribbling on the crackly paper she called onionskin. Reading or writing, she always held a cigarette. "I can't even hear myself think!" she'd exclaim as she shooed the four of us kids out of her sight to play our noisy games somewhere else and leave her alone at the kitchen table.

In one of her downsizings – travelling light she called it – Mom passed on a giant-size plastic storage bin of those letters she wrote to her mother way back when. My grandmother had saved them and given them back, saying they were family history. The bin of letters became a hot potato among my siblings. Steve took the bin first, scanning every page and confident that his new software would search key words. He had no interest in actually reading the letters, though. "It all happened before I was born," he said. When he was done, he passed the bin to Nancy. She became a curator of the collection. Wearing white gloves, she pieced the thousands of random pages together and set them in plastic protectors in date order in nine jumbo-size three-ring binders. "I haven't got time to read them," she said. I knew there was more to it than that as she passed the bin to me. I was excited to get them. I would be the child to mine these artifacts of our family past, seeking understanding I would then share with my siblings. The project went well for a few days until I realized that sadness was building in me. Why did my stomach churn each time I opened a binder? I sought therapy. Over months and hundreds of dollars in fees, I figured out the mystery. Those letters were a nanny camera on our childhoods and where was I? I hungered for references to me, but I was barely mentioned in Mom's relating of her life to her own mother. I appeared in a label: The Twins. Or I was referred to as fat or bossy and it was clear I was not as smart or creative or saintly as anyone else. No wonder I was sad! My therapist recommended that I pack the letters away and get on with my life. They gathered dust in the back of a closet.

"Isn't this nice?" Mom stretched like a cat, pulling back her toes as they touched mine. "We've never had this kind of time, have we?"

"I love to have you all to myself," I answered, trying to hold on to her eyes. She turned away to look at the TV screen. Hours passed. We switched to rum as the shadows grew. I got up to stretch or mix more drinks or empty the ashtray or toss another log on the fire. The millennium show droned on. We were jaded by the endless spectacle. Streams of silk twirled around a thousand dancers somewhere in Asia. Fireworks filled the sky over Beijing. In Africa, a circle of old women, Zulu perhaps, were waving their skinny arms in the air, clapping and bobbing to the beat of drums. "Those babes sure have more zip than I do," Mom said out of our silence. Then, after another pause, came the question that began to shift my world. "Are there old folks' homes in Africa?" What did she want me to say? Was I to connect the dots between these vibrant old ladies and her infirmity encroaching so fast? Or was it just a cultural comment?

I hated old folks' homes and the litany of names that hid their real purpose as warehouses for people whose age had become a burden. Independent living, retirement homes, senior citizen residences, golden-age lodges, assisted-living facilities, nursing homes, long-term care or skilled-nursing facilities. The list of euphemisms seemed endless. However gussied up they were on the outside, inside I felt they housed despair. I told Mom that I guessed South Africa was a generation or two behind us in changes to family life and so old folks' homes would probably be rare. I was more interested in talking about something else. "What happened to your grandmother Rebecca when she got frail?" I asked.

Mom lit another cigarette and puffed for a while as I waited. She said the Great Depression forced her family to move to Halifax when her father lost his job and they were suddenly destitute. Though the old mansion I knew as 2 Mitchell Street was already bursting with other family refugees in despair, Granny Rebecca took them in. Mom said she didn't remember how they shared the space or how the feisty chatelaine of the manor became the frail old lady she tended. The Zulus danced. "Did your Granny Rebecca go to an old folks' home when she dwindled?" I asked.

Mom glared at me with piercing eyes. "Dwindle? What an unkind word for people growing old!" I sensed she wanted to change the subject, but pressed on.

"I don't know, I read it somewhere, and it fits the reality, don't you think?" I explained that dwindling was used in books I read as the description of advancing frailty and unravelling of whatever quality of life was experienced in the early senior years. It was the phase of life when health started to fade but death was still far off. Slow death, perhaps, I mused. "Long time dying isn't the easy way to go, is it?"

Mom's gaze softened. She agreed. Though Granny Rebecca had dwindled, she never saw the inside of an old folks' home. She was the centre of family life, in fact. "It's strange," Mom mused, as she picked a bit of tobacco off the tip of her tongue and crushed another cigarette onto her pile. "It's the creak of her rocker that sticks in my mind." I asked what kind of things she did to help her Granny Rebecca, since in my calculation she must have been under ten years old. "She called me her Little Nurse Betty. That made me proud." The stories began to tumble out and I turned the TV down. The old woman was incontinent and in those days throwaway adult diapers had not been invented. So my child-mother helped my great-grandmother lurch to the outhouse because climbing the stairs to the bathroom was out of the question. Little Nurse Betty spent much of her time cleaning up puddles and wiping her grandmother's bottom. In my childhood, bathroom doors stayed locked, and farting was forbidden. Did Mom's fastidiousness come from that experience? Mom changed the subject.

"Do you know the teacup with the bird on the handle? It was Granny's favorite." I said of course, it was with all the old china in Mom's dining room hutch. "You notice everything." Mom patted my hand, "You are such a good daughter."

What was this flicker of warmth every time I heard the words, 'good daughter'? Did everyone respond as I did to this kind of affirmation? I changed the subject again. "Why didn't your brothers help out?" Mom didn't hesitate. She said that boys and men were bumblers at the job of caregiving. It was a prejudice that I disliked, though I had it a bit myself. I took a different direction.

"Well, did Great-grandma help the family in any way?" Mom said that 2 Mitchell Street was her house, first of all, so she contributed the roof over their heads. I waited while she lit another cigarette and pulled in a lungful of smoke, which she held for a moment while she thought of what else happened in the balance of care and being cared for. She exhaled a cloud. "Potatoes. She spent whole afternoons hacking away at them." Mom said that the smell of peels curling up under the stove at the old woman's feet was a sensory memory for her. Another was the feel of her child toes poking through the holes in her socks. Granny Rebecca knitted furiously but slipped stitches because she couldn't see the wool. No one mentioned it or complained. Knitting gave purpose to the old woman's days. Everyone in the family knew that Granny Rebecca's dignity was as important to her as food. "She never felt like she was a burden," Mom said. "At least she was never a burden to me."

The Zulu crones faded away and now we watched celebrations in Europe: the burning Thames, the Eiffel Tower blazing in fireworks, crowds dancing around the Brandenburg Gate. We watched with half an eye. Mom seemed tired of talking. I was wrong.

"I didn't do right by Alice." This remark had my instant attention. Did that follow from our "being a burden" talk? On the one hand, Granny Rebecca was Mom's dream of perfect dwindling, but on the other, the fading of her own mother, Alice, was her nightmare. Tears welled up in Mom's eyes and I wordlessly shoved the box of tissues her way. She scrunched several and dabbed. A wad of regret, I thought. "But I had no choice," she said in a low and wavering voice.

That was the nub of it. In one generation, the norms around elder care had changed.

We reminisced about how we wrenched my grandmother from Halifax against her will, more than a decade before. The details had faded in my mind but the traumatic feelings were still fresh. I had been juggling my overflowing inbox the day when the phone rang and it was Mom. She was crying. I knew there was trouble because she had never called me at work before. Mom was in her own office in Calgary. I called it her corner office and it was far fancier than mine in Ottawa. She was a top manager of her training organization, I was just one of the crowd in my midsize government department. I heard my mother's desperation. She explained how my grandmother, Alice, a woman in her eighties barely managing in her bedsit apartment yet proud of her independence, had just been evicted. There had been one burned pot on the stove too many, too many fights with the neighbours, and any sympathy or help from her Halifax relatives had dried up. My Aunt Clare, living just a neighbourhood away from her mother, not across the continent like Mom did, had turned her back completely. Some Maritimer feud, Mom said, I couldn't possibly understand. But Alice had crossed the line in her assisted-living apartment, and she was out on her ear. In this crisis, Aunt Clare refused to even answer the phone calls from her mother's facility. Instead, Clare had called Mom, her sister, and insisted it was her turn to be the daughter-caregiver. Mom said there had been a doozy of a long-distance argument until Clare had just hung up on her. Mom knew that Clare was right. It was up to her to look after Alice now. She'd got off easy through all these dwindling years. Along with rational acceptance of this, Mom was consumed by guilt.

"I need you," Mom had said to me. "I can't do this move alone."

8

I thought about how I would take time off at this busy time in my job and manage my family, too, dropping everything and flying to Halifax. Even as I was making these instant calculations, I said, "OK, I'll meet you in Grandma's apartment."

"You are such a good daughter," Mom replied. Two days later, both of us dead tired, Mom and I hugged hello in the sad scorched kitchen of my grandmother. Alice rocked in her chair looking dazed and tired. Mutely, she watched Mom and me press on through that awful day of packing up a life. We didn't speak as we grimly sorted her world into garbage bags marked donate or trash. We stuffed the essentials into two oversize suitcases to take to Calgary. That night, as Mom and I slept in exhaustion on the lumpy pull out sofa, Grandma unpacked everything. "You can't make me go!" she screamed the next morning when we woke up bleary-eyed to see her clothes back in her closet, her Bible and lives of the saints on her bedside table and the china dogs she loved back on the shelf where they had been the day before. "This is my home, I hate Calgary," she wailed. We ignored her pleas as we started over. Finally, the three of us were at the airport with Grandma in a wheelchair. Clare and her family had come to say goodbye. She was grim as she offered her mother one stiff hug and a kiss on the wrinkled rouged cheek. Then she hissed to Mom, "Good riddance." I thought how difficult it must have been for Clare all those years, trying to support her mother, and how sad and lonely my grandmother must have been, with her growing dependence on a hostile daughter. I could not understand how or why Grandma's support system had become so tattered. I just knew that it was better for my grandmother to be in Calgary now. But how would

Mom manage to care for Grandma and love her, while holding onto the job she also loved? In her suburban three-bedroom home, Mom crowded Grandma into the tiny guest room with the shared bathroom down the hall. She hired neighbours to stay with the old lady while she struggled to stay on top of her job, and also be there for her husband and her teenaged sons. No home help Mom hired lasted more than a month or two before Alice sent them packing. "Quit your job, Betty!" her mother pleaded. "Be with me. I need you." Mom became hardened to my grandmother's desperation, perhaps in denial that the situation was unravelling. "You are not a good daughter," Alice raged. Mom's boss finally said something needed to change on the home front, or she would need to pass her files to someone else who could give the job more attention. But the corner office was the pinnacle of all Mom's dreams. So when a colleague passed on a tip about a space opening in a nursing home on Mom's route between her home and office, she grabbed the chance to put Grandma away. Mom was convinced that she had no choice. In my secret self where I kept my harsh opinions, I felt Mom had made a selfish decision. But even so, I had to admit that Alice did need more help than Mom could ever provide. And Mom visited every day.

I visited Grandma once, too. I was shocked to see her buckled into a Geri-Chair that engulfed her shriveled body. She huddled behind a curtain that separated her from three other old ladies sharing the room. The crucifix above Grandma's grey metal hospital bed featured a hangdog Jesus whose suffering seemed no greater than Grandma's was. I'd weaved my way to her cubbyhole past carts piled high with diapers, lines of wheelchairs occupied by bewildered oldsters, and staff who didn't smile. There was bedlam as thready voices called

10

out for help and bells jangled, unnoticed, it seemed. I gagged on the smell of antiseptic, fried food, and old urine. I couldn't bear to stay with my grandmother for long. She didn't know me, anyway. I never returned. She died a few months later. My repulsion toward nursing homes as the right thing to do went back to that traumatic time. Now, with the fire dying to embers, and both of us worn down by the emotion of these memories, Mom said she needed a nap. I needed a rest, too.

Like I always did when I felt restless, I phoned my twin in Calgary. Judi was preoccupied with Dad, not sad old memories of dwindling. It was his wedding day. In the last ten minutes before midnight, my father would ask a woman we barely knew to stick by him for better or worse, in sickness and in health, as long as they both would live. I was still amazed at the thought that Martha would actually say, "I do."

"He's telling everyone that Martha is his tax strategy," Judi chuckled. "He says he'll save a bundle because she'll be a deduction for all of 1999 but won't cost him a nickel." I laughed, too. I asked if he was pressuring Martha. Judi didn't think so. Martha had confided to her that Dad was twisting her arm but she was driving a hard bargain in return. We knew the deal. Martha would be his caregiver with privileges. In exchange, Dad would provide the financial security she needed. In Martha, Dad had found the solution to his end-of-life care needs. In Fred, this stranger who became my stepmother had found her sugar daddy.

Hours later, after midnight had come and gone in Ottawa, we talked again. I asked her how she was doing in all the kerfuffle of the nuptials. "You really do get me," Judi marvelled. "Everyone else just wants me to talk about what's up with Dad. But not you." She reminded me, with what I heard over the phone lines as a gag of emotion, that no one was closer to her than I was. Judi and I shared twin souls that only we could really understand. The rest of that first night of the century, I restlessly tossed in bed, thinking of Dad and Mom. Dad had his care plan figured out. Mom did not. My great-grandmother Rebecca had died in her own bed in that period between the world wars, in the centre of family life. Ten years ago, her daughter and my Grandmother Alice had died of loneliness in a nursing home. Now Alice's daughter, my mother, was next in this sequence of the generations. How would I respond when my turn came to be the caregiving daughter?

By dawn I knew. I called it my millennium vow and gave it a name that fit the way I knew how to run things, 'The Parent Project'. Whatever challenges lay ahead with Mom and Dad, I would support them. I felt relief in a nagging decision now made, and strength of purpose for the way ahead. "I'm in if you are," Judi said when I told her of my resolution. We both knew it was a commitment that would engage us in ways we could not yet imagine. She would be Daughter on Deck, and bear the brunt of what care was needed for Mom and Dad day-to-day. I would be Daughter at a Distance, since I lived so far away. I'd have her back, though, and be fully engaged with it all. We were going to be the twin team, entwined in the years ahead, and that thought gave us joy.

Mom and I had a few more days left in this visit. Mom just wanted more time to laze on the sofa, drinking coffee and rum and playing occasional Scrabble while we talked. I was hungry for her stories of how I came to be. I ransacked old pictures from unsorted piles. We steeped ourselves in stories triggered by the memories revealed in these artifacts like some

12

family archaeology. Finally, it was time for her to go back to Calgary. Our hugs good-bye seemed more intimate than they had been before. I knew something was different, though I had no idea what the future would bring. Still, those three days were the crucible of what became my caregiving story.

2

The Way We Were

"Never let the truth ruin a good story."

History was tricky to Mom. She loved mysteries where real people in the Middle Ages had unbelievable adventures. She scoffed at anyone who looked for too much truth in stories. What mattered was a different kind of honesty, the version of truth that probed what lay beneath the facts. When it came to family history, what actually happened was only part of the way we were.

We snuggled under the blanket, no longer pulling our toes away when they touched. She told me how John went to get her medicine when I was an embryo and making her nauseous. I listened without a challenge. Of course no two-year-old could ride the bus to the Hudson's Bay downtown with a note pinned to his shirt to pick up her anti-vomiting pills. That was obviously false. But the reality of her emotion about John, her saintly toddler, was spot on. I did want to probe beneath her truth, though. For example, how did the unlikely couple of Betty Abraham and Fred Perry manage to forge the relationship that became my family? Her recollections of early marriage were grim. Or what secrets in her past made Mom become the patient sufferer now, dismissing discomfort with her favorite phrase, 'It is what it is'? Saying that, she still managed to convey her pain in body language, and phrases like, "Don't you worry" or "I'm offering it up for the souls in purgatory." And what about Dad? Could she tell me what she knew of his childhood? How had he become a happy-go-lucky optimist who shut down us kids when we whined with, "Stop your belly-aching!" How did he learn to manipulate? That was the part of Dad that Mom detested the most. I put another log on the fire and poked it till the flames took over. Where could I begin? "What do you know about when you were born?" I asked. Birth stories were significant, I knew. Mine was. They were sometimes precursors of what would unfold later in life. Did hers hold clues? Mom smiled as she lit a cigarette from the stub of the one before, and began.

"Well, I almost didn't get born at all!" she began. Obviously the story was secondhand but it was the first truth of her life. Her parents battled furiously all the time, though they stayed together as a good Catholic family getting the parenting job done. Five kids through the great Depression and an awful war. But this job was getting Mom safely into the world. Mom had been told it was a particularly icy day in the middle of January 1923. She knew my grandmother's contractions started strong and just got worse and closer together, but there was a Maritime blizzard blowing. Alice bundled her toddler boys against the cold and carried them through the snowstorm to the neighbour, while my grandfather tried to clear his rum-soaked brain and hitch the reluctant horse to the sleigh. Together they headed out through the blizzard to the rural hospital, fighting fear and the disorienting gusts of wind. Grandma screamed all the way, hurling abuse at my grandfather, Mom said, but that was conjecture, too. The fact was, they arrived just in time to the tiny Cape Breton case room with my mother crowning and then slithering into the world without further fuss. Other than her near miss of being born on a sleigh, Mom's infancy was unremarkable. "There was so much shouting in my childhood," she said, "that I made a vow never to raise my voice to you kids." It was true that I had no memory as a child of being yelled at. She used other tactics to get her anger across. But that was another story.

Mom was named Rebecca after her grandmother, but she never liked the name. Rebecca Elizabeth Abraham sounded Jewish. So when she could, she changed that. Rebecca became Elizabeth Therese at her confirmation. St. Therese was her absolute favorite saint. She had a collection of medals, holy cards, prayers to Therese, who was also called the Little Flower. The part Mom liked best about the Little Flower was that she became a nun barely through adolescence. Hers was a special vocation, Mom said, of contemplation and prayer in silence for the rest of her days. What a life! Mom envied it, she said, and told me how she tried to join a convent when she was in her teens. She was winding up for that story but I interrupted her. I didn't want her to get waylaid into telling me about my spiritual starvation.

"What is the first thing you remember?" I waited while Mom blew her nose and lit another cigarette.

"I fell on a glass and tore my face to shreds." She felt her chin for the scar that had always been invisible to everyone else. Toddler Betty had been running away from a spanking that day in 1925. She'd done something she couldn't remember, of course, but since it was a crystal glass that drove into her face that day, she surmised she was in a childish game of catch me. She remembered blood everywhere. She also could feel in memory her mother's hysteria, screaming at her to stop fussing. The country doctor put in 26 stitches, Mom said. The phrase that echoed down through Mom's life after that, her mother's attempt to calm her then, was, "It doesn't hurt." Was that the x factor that made Mom so stoic in life? Mom didn't know. But one thing she believed was that those scars meant she was flawed in a family that admired beauty. Clare was the pretty child. Mom became the smart one. She read a book or more a day in the constantly-page-turning manner that always fascinated me and made me envious.

Mom wanted to follow in the steps of the Little Flower, but Clare beat her to the punch. Her sister joined a convent but was kicked out before she took any vows. When Mom said she had a vocation, too, her mother raged. "I will not be shamed again." So Mom gave up that dream and reset her goals to become a teacher instead.

But war was brewing. Halifax filled with soldiers. After years of unemployment in the Great Depression, her father was working again. His job was secret, in the Royal Naval Shipyards in Dartmouth. He had the skills of a cable operator, so Mom surmised it had something to do with communications. The future was frightening but day-to-day life in pre-war Halifax was upbeat. Mom said that coming of age in that time trained her to focus on the present and not worry about what might come around the next bend.

When my grandfather bragged to his senior officer about his whiz-kid daughter and her photographic memory, Mom was asked to an interview and then encouraged to join the war effort as a code maker and breaker. Mom said she liked the job, except for its requirement for secrecy. Telling me this, she paused to stub out her cigarette and reach for another.

"Can you tell me more about your work in espionage?"
I knew we had left Mom's comfort zone now, but pressed on.
It had been some years before when she had revealed being
a spy. It was her 70th birthday, and she was cutting her cake
when she said she had a confession. I remembered how agitated she had been that day as she told us, her adult children,
about this secret life. "Just talking about makes me feel like a
traitor," she said that day, but insisted it was OK, the Official
Secrets Act had been repealed. "I'm tired of keeping it all
inside." We were thrilled to discover our James Bond mother,
and pumped her for more details. She'd gone silent, though,
saying those memories made her sad. "I want to celebrate my
life now. Imagine! I'm seventy!" She changed the subject and
refused our urging to say more. Now I saw my chance.

"I was not a spy, dear," she began. "It was Naval Intelligence." She explained that she was getting ready for University
when the order came. She was told to join the Halifax Infirmary as a student nurse instead. In this role, she would get
close to the victims of the torpedo attacks in the wards where
they were taken when their battered bodies were fished out of
the North Atlantic. Most casualties of the Battle of the Atlantic were merchant marines in the supply convoys, but some
were sailors from all over the place, including Germany. The
U-boat submarine survivors were patched up in the Infirmary,
too, before being moved into prisoner-of-war camps if they
survived. Mom spoke high-school German. She became the
gentle interrogator and witness to every word and tortured
cry. Where were they headed when they were hit? How did
they know where the convoys would be? She mopped their
brows, scraped the rot off their stumps, and robbed them of
their secrets. The next morning before class, she passed all

the bits of information up the line. Mom was a great nurse, and an even more effective secret agent. But it blew her mind apart. She had her first nervous breakdown before she was twenty. The nuns who ran the Infirmary had no patience for such weakness and no idea about her covert traumas. When she would not stop sobbing, Mom was sent home to 2 Mitchell Street to the care of her mother. My grandmother had no time for a sniveling daughter. She said she was ashamed of her and put Mom to work scrubbing all the floors and washing the walls and then doing it over and over. Soap on, soap off. "Get a grip," was my grandmother's only advice. Mom did, but the theme of suffering in silence ran through her psyche forevermore.

And Dad? His father died between one day and the next of the Spanish Flu, before my baby-parent was walking. Loss rocked his world before he'd truly entered it. He talked about Boy Scout bliss, Mom said, valuing those experiences more than any other. Mom said his brothers were bullies and his sister a nut case, so he was a lonely child. His mother was a miser. She kept an account of every penny she spent on Fred, and presented it to him the day he graduated with an engineering degree from Queens. Eventually, she removed him from her will. He'd married a papist, according to Mom, and was breeding like a rabbit. Mom said she hated her mother-in-law. I had only one memory, of the old lady lying stiff and forbidding in her upscale nursing home. Dad lined us kids up, oldest to youngest, to be introduced. "Kiss your Granny," he commanded. "She loves you." I did. She stared at me wordlessly with gummy eyes, her paper lips not kissing me back.

As a kid, Dad embarrassed me. He dragged me every Saturday to the back of stores like Safeway to have a talk with his buddy, the produce manager. "Is there anything headed to the trash that you can give to me? You, know, bananas turning black, bruised apples, wilted veggies?" He pointed to us, his hungry children. We peered silently back at the man. Then Dad turned us loose in the grocery, hunting for dented cans that he could get a deal on, too. I was five or six then and learning the uses of guilt. Even then I felt the shame of seeing people smirk. If Dad was embarrassed, he never gave a hint. Mom said he couldn't see past what he needed people to do for him. Her life with Fred was one long humiliation, she said.

"How did you two get together, then?"

"That's a story that goes better with rum!" Mom said she didn't care if it wasn't noon yet. Neither did I. I mixed the first drink of the day, seeing it as lubricant for her memories that might cast light on mine. Mom smacked her lips as she sipped the rum, warming now to her chronicle of marital calamity.

Betty caught Fred's eye immediately at the navy dance where they met. Dad's gang of cocky civilians was cutting in on Mom's gang of student nurses and sailors. Mom smiled. "I was not impressed from the first moment I met your father." He jitterbugged well, she admitted, but added he was a braggart and a dandy who had no insight about how boring he really was. To her, at least, she admitted. Mom's girlfriends loved Freddie. At least they loved his Model T and the shack he owned with friends from the oil refinery where he worked producing the fuel for the war machine. The cottage was beside a weedy lake filled with leeches, Mom recalled. Still, it was far enough into the country that it was an ideal getaway for weekend parties and from the stresses of Halifax. No way would Mom's friends let her jilt Freddie and their ticket out of town. But when Dad proposed, Mom said no. The fib she told was her big mistake. She said she loved him, of course she did, but how could she marry him, since he was not a Catholic? "I thought that got me off the hook," Mom said, lighting a cigarette from the nub of the one before. "But your father had no scruples about that, either." In secret he took the set of lessons he needed to learn how to be a Catholic and then be baptized. That same day, he revealed his subterfuge to Mom, sly but still so needy. "He said I must marry him now, because he had made this huge sacrifice to win me." Mom took a last gulp of rum and swirled the ice in the bottom of her glass, holding it out for a refill. "What a cad!"

As I dutifully mixed another drink in the kitchen, I thought about all this and felt torn. If that was the way Mom remembered it, then for sure, Dad was a sneak. But wasn't Mom also a liar? Hadn't she manipulated him just as much as he had used her? I knew I must keep my mouth shut, though. Those would be fighting words. She would say she was tired of talking, say she had a headache, say she needed a nap. She would freeze me out, and that fear always held me back from too much honesty. I passed her the fresh rum and she sipped it. "Then what?" I asked.

Mom conceived John on her wedding night and vomited into every ditch along the honeymoon road. The tender trap clamped shut with the first baby and stayed that way through six more children. They endured their partnership for forty years, doing all the things that couples of the fifties and sixties did to raise a Catholic brood. They never achieved harmony, though, and we kids never felt the warmth of their marital affection. None of us were surprised when the marriage came apart as soon as they felt free of their obligations as parents to us.

Dad was an oilman. Calgary was the booming oil town. They moved west just after the war, with me in utero, and landed in a housing crisis. My first home was in an attic squat, rented for $35 a month from a widow who was mentally ill. She raised budgie birds, and kept their cages in the only bathtub. Her bulldog was trained to use the one toilet. Everything about Mom's early married life was terrible, she said, except for John. Mom would have found her life perfect if motherhood had stopped with him. But that was not the Catholic way. "I did my wifely duty," Mom sighed. I said I was glad. It meant I was born. That is what I really wanted to know about.

"Tell me about my birth."

According to Mom, Dad's first question when she said she was pregnant with me was to probe whether ending it was an option. He only said that once, though, she admitted. The first secret of my life was that there were two of us starting our twin journey, not one embryo. From that first split egg, Judi and I grew so tightly bound to each other that to Dr. Gibson we felt like one. When we were ready to be born, eight weeks premature, a student nurse heard two heartbeats. Mom's braggart bumbler doctor scoffed. Mom's belly was too small even for one baby. But the student nurse was right. I smiled to imagine the smug look on her face when my thatch of hair began to peek out of the now bloody portal opened by Judi's arrival. But as I appeared, Judi stole the show by dying. At least that's how it seemed. She'd been laid on the metal table beside Mom's head while the focus was on me, and so only Mom noticed that this tiny infant was not breathing. She didn't really get it that this was her baby, though. In her gas-induced waking dream, she thought the dead fetus, blue and rigid on the table beside her head, was from some other unfortunate mother. Dr. Gibson took one look at Judi and shrieked. The focus shifted off me struggling to take my first breath, to pump more air into my twin. I guessed that was my first compromise. I had needs, but hers were bigger. They mattered more.

I weighed four pounds and some ounces, and Judi much less. Even together we were not up to the average weight of one full-term baby. Mom's fear was not that we would die, though everyone knew this was a likely outcome. She was afraid that our little souls would languish in limbo for eternity if she didn't act fast. Mom demanded a priest. The dribble of holy water on our still-bloody heads saved us from that fate before we were an hour old. "What do you want to call them," the priest asked, staring at us new Catholics naked in our preemie dishpan under a heat lamp. "Call them both Mary," Mom said. "We'll sort it out if they live."

For the next six weeks Twin 1 and Twin 2 clutched each other in a single plastic bassinet. I didn't want Mom to get started on Dad in this account of my early infancy. She had told me plenty of times before how he said a quick hello before he said goodbye and flew off to Toronto on a business trip. Later Mom learned about Lavinia and realized that Dad had left us dying for a tryst. Once home, though, Mom admitted that Dad was key to our early survival. "He was the milkman." She said we couldn't breastfeed because we had no suck reflexes and, anyway, her breasts were so infected that her milk oozed from open sores. These were the days before premixed baby formula, so Dr. Gibson said to try whey, the sour liquid left over from making cheese. We might be able to digest it better than cow's milk. Dad hung around the back door of the Alpha Dairy every morning to get that by-product before it was thrown away. That freebie saved our lives.

After eight weeks, I beat Judi home and took up residence in a drawer lined with hot water bottles. For a few weeks I was the apple of everyone's eye. When Judi made survival weight, Mom fell apart, she admitted. "You were already too much to handle. How could I manage two?"

Mom's memories of her twins in the first months were hazy. There was a howling dog, and through the first early spring icicles formed on John's crib set up in the closed, but not insulated, verandah. Frost was thick on all the windows from the hot moisture of the kettle kept boiling to add humidity and help us breathe. Mom tied a blue bow on Judi's toe so that visitors would not be confused, but soon that was not needed. I began life a pound heavier than Judi – that was a third bigger – and stayed pudgy. People began to call me "the fat twin."

"What is your first memory, by the way?" Mom asked. She said she wanted to listen for a while. It was my turn to share a story.

"Jealousy. I think my first memory is jealousy," I began after a long pause.

Judi had an anger problem from an early age. When Mom heard about a newfangled idea called child psychiatry she was all for trying it out on her unhappy five-year-old. So every week for a year we all trooped downtown to the Child Guidance Clinic: John, Judi, Nancy and me. While Mom flipped through magazines and Nancy coloured and John read his easy-reader book, I stewed. Every time Judi came bouncing out of her session with a report of knocking down towers or pulling the heads off dolls with penises, I was insane with envy. Why wasn't I getting to do this, too? Judi was having fun and I was not. Was I a bad twin?

"I should have explained it better to you, but you never complained." Mom pulled the blanket to her chin and tickled my toes with hers. "Both of you were always a joy to me. You are good daughters."

Puberty tore Judi and me apart as we struggled for separateness. We rejected being twinned. Judi stretched a rope down the middle of the room we shared, our little Iron Curtain. At seventeen, our rivalry peaked. Judi was leaving home because she couldn't stand Mom anymore, and Mom was letting her go because the feeling was mutual. I wanted to escape, too, but I knew there was no way. Mom said she needed me to help her with the housework and look after my baby brothers, so she could get on with her own life plan. Another nervous breakdown had undone her, and the cure appeared to be that she must follow her dream at last and go to university. I was consumed with sorrow about the imminent parting from my twin, but since we were enemies, I could not show my feelings. Instead, while Judi learned to ski moguls with friends I did not have, I stayed home and learned to knit. Now, in the last month of the last summer together, I was stitching all my pain into a warm wool sweater for Judi. It was my parting gift, my peace offering, my statement of love. Judi didn't know the sweater was for her. She mocked me for being so prissy, said I was a real loser not having a gang like she did. One day, when the gift was almost complete, I came to my side of the room and found the floor knee deep in a curly forest of green wool. My eyes widened in shock. "It's a stupid sweater," Judi hissed, her eyes squinting through her cat's eye frames with a look of malice. "I did you a favor getting rid of it."

25

"Yeah? Well, it was for you...you stupid creep, I was making a sweater for you!" My own myopic eyes filled with tears as Judi's grew wide with shock. Then we both burst into simultaneous sobs, kicking aside the rope between us and the tangle of wool. We clung to each other with our choked apologies. I guessed it was the moment we both grew up.

The demands of husbands, families and careers meant physical distance through our adulthood, but we stayed heart-close. People still said they couldn't tell us apart. We knew it was uncanny how we could finish each other's sentences, just as we had done as little girls. Judi called me when I went into labour with my first child, saying she wondered what was up because cramps were driving her insane. We were never surprised to have the same dream. We dressed alike when we could. Though I was two inches taller and ten pounds heavier, we maintained exactly the same Body Mass Index. Both Judi and I meant it when we said, "She's my other half." We didn't need to become a tight team to pull off the Parent Project. We already were.

3

Need Creep

"I'm making my own decisions!"

Judi and I called it 'need creep'. Anyone observing Mom living alone in her upscale condo in downtown Calgary and going out with the girls to the theatre, or Dad in the suburbs with Martha, would have seen two elderly people in vigorous old age. That was a facade. Behind it, Judi was making them both look good. Emails between us became threads of irritation some days, and vague sadness on others. Still, we were always problem-solving as we worked through how we could make things better for Mom one day and Dad the next. It might be how to change a light bulb on a high ceiling, or fix a running toilet, or how to get past both Mom and Dad's fear of television remotes. We were both frustrated by Dad's inability to work his phone message machine. Dad said no one wanted to talk to him as he shouted at the recorded messages. He could not understand the role of the blinking light on the phone. Finally, we figured out that the only way to soothe Dad was to make cleaning the messages a job of any family visitor. Computerized banking was beyond both of them, but Dad was also terrified of automatic teller machines. They would eat his card for sure. When credit cards required

27

passwords, Judi wrote his secret number inside his hatband. He kept forgetting where he put it. But Judi insisted she didn't mind being the financial and legal assistant to Mom and Dad. She said they were grateful to the point of embarrassment. She monitored their investments and kept contact with their advisers. She helped them bundle their receipts and get them to the accountants she trusted at tax time. She sat with them to update their wills. She figured out the differences between all the powers of attorney, for finances and for personal care. Reluctantly, she took on the job as executor. "Just in case I die," Dad said. After Judi took a course to learn the ropes of this, she phoned me to say she was full of foreboding. Dwindling was not easy. Death would be worse.

From my home across the Rocky Mountains and a stretch of Pacific Ocean, I bumped up Judi's spirits when they flagged, and was her always-willing ear. She minimized all the hours spent here and there, berating herself when she complained, but admitting I had a point when I told her it all added up to a part-time personal assistant job on top of her other one. That was the real rub. Judi's career depended on using those hours she spent as the go-to girl to earn real pay. She worried about where her career was headed. She loved being her own boss, and the creative work she did so well. But working from home was hazardous. "Mom and Dad think I'm just sitting back peeling grapes around here when they ask me to do something for them. They don't know I have to put off something else I'm getting paid for." It was true. Mom and Dad saw her as always able to take them to an appointment or join them in some pleasure that was only really fun for them, or possible, with her company and help. Judi moaned that she was losing her edge in a competitive field. Inevitably Judi knew she was perceived as less able to deliver a project in a tight deadline than the other bidders, and she lost contracts she would have snapped up in the days before the Parent Project. At those times of Judi's despair my job was to flood her psyche with my sympathy.

I tried to be the social convener for Mom and Dad when I came to Calgary, so that Judi could say with honesty, "Just wait till Janet gets here – then we'll have some real fun!"

On every visit, Dad invited me to his community church. At coffee hour he glowed, introducing me around to all the same buddies he had introduced me to the last time. It hurt me to watch them glance at us as we approached, Dad grinning and telling me how I would love to meet so-and-so, and then see so-and-so move away to avoid this rambling man. When cornered, they said Fred was at the centre of everything at First Lutheran. I figured I had a role to add a few more stories to the mix and maybe give them all more to talk about with Dad when I wasn't there.

Supporting Mom's social life was more complicated but a lot more fun. When I was growing up, the daughter who was stuck at home, her parties for foreign students studying at the university were legendary. I loved to watch her leading the dancing at Perry Party Central where there were so many afros bobbing to reggae beats that the beams supporting the floor boards of the family room began to buckle. Then Mom brought out the grub. Forty pounds of paella cooked in pots meant for canning pickles, and gone in a flash, leaving the sounds of lips smacking and the sight of chicken bones everywhere for me to pick up afterwards. These bonanzas were her happy time. They ruled her self-image still, though she was out of gas even to produce a dinner for two. I knew how party time made Mom glow, and that was all I needed to suggest throwing one when I came to visit. In truth, Judi and I enjoyed them too. Judi led the brainstorming, fuelled by rum, as we decided on the theme of each party. Robbie Burns met Chinese New Year once. Everything was plaid and wontons were on the menu along with haggis. Another time, we celebrated the Olympics with all the old gear from 1988, the event Calgary never forgot. Everyone wore a red scarf and we ate hot dogs. One other afternoon we served tea and told fortunes. Mom's contribution to planning was to smile with pleasure and dictate a list of invitees. Mine was to do the shopping and what cooking was needed. On the morning of a party, Mom always woke up saying she was sore with no zip at all and could I please cancel it? I always refused, and Mom would sit wanly watching me work, but come to life with the first ring of the doorbell. Afterwards Mom glowed for days as compliments flowed in from guests who wondered how Mom did it. "The twins helped me a little bit," she would admit.

The truth was, neither Mom nor Dad appreciated Judi's ministrations. Dad tasked her with the phrase she detested, an offhand, "Oh, by the way, I have a problem." His false teeth were loose so it came out as 'pwablem'. Mom framed her job lists as a favor since otherwise, what else would Judi be doing? And Mom could be catty. Behind her back, she whined how Judi kowtowed to her husband's parents, and how she spoiled her grandsons, and didn't Dad have that woman Martha to keep him company? Why did he need to pester Judi? When Judi and I settled down in our respective time zones for a beer and a bellyache, the topic was always the same. Judi never felt she was able to do enough. Did she see the need creep, as I did? I told her the story of the boiled frog. It was a simple parable about a frog winding up somehow in a pot of cold water placed over a fire. The water got hotter. The frog adapted one degree at a time, not even thinking about hopping out to save itself, till of course it stewed to its death. If any other frog put one toe in the pot it leapt out of danger, pronto. Judi rejected this metaphor. She wasn't the boiled frog. She just found comfort in complaining and it was my job to listen, not tell her what to do. Most of the time she got a kick out of being Daughter on Deck. Like Mom, she was a Scrabble fan. Like Mom, she loved watching a movie from Blockbuster or following a reality show on TV. Like Dad, she enjoyed walking along the river. She was sorry for whining, Judi always said after one of these conversations. Forget it. She was fine.

On one visit to Calgary, I saw big signs in the parking lot across the street from Mom's high-rise condo. An assisted-living facility was in the works. Mom was disgusted about it at first. It would block her view of the mountains. I wondered aloud, though, if she might like to move to Bow Claire when it was ready, and get her view back. "Skate to where the puck is headed, eh, Mom?" I said. Sooner or later, Mom would need more help. Why not get settled in before that time came? I suggested that on my next visit we could take a tour of the show suite.

"OK, just to please you," Mom said. A few months later we took a tour. "Wow!" was Mom's first reaction, "they allow smokers!" That was rare now, and Mom knew it. She would never give up her habit of a lifetime though she admitted the world was making her feel like a pariah now. "But the kitchens? Did you see how tiny they are?" I knew that was a deal breaker. How could she put together dinner parties with a two-burner stove and no oven? "Nope, Bow Claire is not my cup of tea," Mom said. She insisted she was managing fine, though, with just a hand from Judi now and again. I shrugged and let the matter drop. "Have it your way, Mom, it's your decision." I realized how deeply her identity was wired into making meals to feed a crowd. There were so many losses in getting old. She didn't need to add the loss of a kitchen.

Our visits went both ways. I went to Calgary. They visited me on the Coast. I invited them often, one after the other, of course. There could be no more together times after their divorce. They stayed a couple of weeks each time. My husband noted that Mom and Dad seemed to enjoy thinking about their visits more than the real thing. Dad insisted that he loved hiking all the old-growth forest trails. In truth, he would stagger for a few meters down a chip path and then say he was cold. For most of his time he dozed in the recliner, looking out at the woods from beside the fire. And Mom? She thrilled at the smell of the sea when she first arrived. But the closest she got to the ocean was when we parked in French Creek harbor and she watched the fishing boats go in and out. After a cigarette or two, she was ready to head back to her recliner by the fire, and CNN. Mom came to the Coast more often. Dad and Martha were busy with seniors-only bus trips. But eventually Martha admitted they had been asked not to sign up for any more of those. Dad snored loudly as soon as he got on the bus. He took too long to stagger from A to B. Other seniors were getting annoyed and shunning Dad. But Martha was not about to stop the tours just because Dad was not welcome. She was enjoying life and his family would just have to look after her husband when she took a solo holiday. Dad admitted he would also welcome a break from his loquacious bride.

Once Judi came to visit on the Coast at the same time Dad did. It was a surprise. We decided to play our favorite twin trick on Dad, the one we called, "Is it Judi or Janet?" Everyone in on the joke giggled with anticipation at the switch as Judi and I dressed in the same jeans and red sweatshirts and fluffed our same shade of hair in the same direction. Then Dad and I settled side by side to watch the six o'clock news program that was a big part of his day. Half way through I excused myself to go to the bathroom, and Judi slipped into my chair, stifling her giggles. My husband Ed got the camera ready. "Surprise!" I said, leaping back into the room with my arms thrown wide for a group hug. Dad looked at Judi beside him. His face registered confusion and then crumpled. His voice was strangled. "Are you Janet then? Who is Judi then? Where am I then? Are you a twin then?" I guessed our trick triggered the thing Dad feared the most, forgetting his family. My heart grew cold with my own dismay. What were we thinking, toying with Dad's mind? Even if that brain exasperated me sometimes, it was the part of my father that was most endearing. Now it was showing those first tangles of the trouble that lay ahead. Dad hid his chagrin in a wild temper. You are bad daughters was the gist of his rant, tricksters, while Judi and I blushed and stammered our apologies. Silence descended on the rest of the news and into the nature program beyond. Dad recovered his good cheer. We pretended that the incident had not happened. I vowed never to pull a stunt like that again. All of us knew now what Martha had been saying about Dad for months but we had denied. There was no more doubt. Dad was in early dementia.

We did try, however, to work around this new weakness. My husband went with him to visit his relatives in New York. So that Dad didn't feel he was being chaperoned, we told him how much we admired his generosity in letting his freeloading son-in-law come along for the ride. When Nancy invited him to Vancouver, we told Dad we wanted to go too. Would he let us? He loved the trip but couldn't figure out what city he was in or what the event was that had brought us there. Still, for a while it seemed important to make what concessions were needed to protect a key part of Dad's identity: Fred the travelling man.

The seven Perry kids as adults lived all over the country and indeed the world, but we made one commitment. We would move mountains to be together at big events: birthdays with a zero or a five for Mom and Dad, and all the weddings of our own kids. That's how we all wound up in a dark bar the Sunday morning after my nephew Ryan's wedding. Everyone nursed a Starbucks and some of my siblings nursed a hangover. We were gathered for a family meeting. Judi and I were tired from the night before. No one but Judi and I had been aware of Mom's tension building at the reception as wine made Dad bold and he pestered Judi to bring him to Mom's table for a chat and to introduce his new wife. Judi knew there would be a scene, and so the two of us had schemed all evening to keep them apart. Afterwards, debriefing in the room we shared on the other side of the connecting door from Mom, we laughed at ourselves for caring. Wasn't their feud, fulminating for more than half a century, really their business? We agreed it was not our job to protect them from themselves. Still, we felt the task we called peacekeeping was important. It protected the faux tranquility that all the rest of us valued.

The family meeting had one item on the agenda. Should Mom move into Judi's apartment building and live just seven floors below her, rather than across town? "I will make my own decisions," Mom said, "but I want to see what you children think." She said she had decided against assisted living. Bow Claire was too expensive and too small and had no kitchen. Anyway, she just needed a little bit of help from time to time. With Judi upstairs, things would be easier for both of them. Judi wouldn't have to cross town to be with her as she did now and Mom could share her car with Judi. It would be a 50-50 arrangement of caring for each other. We all knew the real question, though. Would this new proximity make things easier for Judi or infinitely more challenging? The discussion went around the room, all of us choosing our words carefully. Then it was John's turn to say his piece.

"It is a lousy idea," he said. Everyone stiffened. Intellectually John was beyond compare. Emotionally, he could be dumb. Mom lit another cigarette, paying no attention to the no smoking signs around the room. "It is a bad idea to be too close to Judi. She is at risk of becoming co-dependent." John looked around the room at all of us, fixing on what eyes would meet his. "She may be that already. I'm concerned for her well-being." There was still silence, so he went on to explain that being across town Judi still could choose whether or not to respond to the needs that would certainly start to grow. In his parish work as a priest, he saw too often how well-intentioned caregiving became something toxic for everyone involved. This thing he called co-dependence happened when being helpful to someone who was essentially competent shifted and became taking on more than was needed or wanted. It robbed confidence from the person being helped. It became an addiction to being needed in the person doing the helping. As generous as it seemed on the outside, there was nothing good about co-dependence. It was dysfunction, pure and simple. The only sound in the room now was the slurping of coffee. Was John winding up for one of his sermons or did he just not know when it was time to shut up? He had more to say. Daughters were most affected by co-dependence. "They learn early that putting everyone else first is the right way to be. The family teaches that."

Next move, Mom. What would she say? Did she feel challenged that she might be turning Judi and me into emotional cripples? Tension rippled through the room. My brother Chris broke the strain. He had a special way of doing that. A half smile. A shrug. And then a pointed question, the kind no one else would dare to ask. He faced John. "What are you talking about?" He said it all sounded flaky to him. And besides, he figured Judi liked being the one in charge of things. I glanced furtively around the room. How was everyone else taking this? John sat leaning forward, his legs crossed and arms folded. Judi had her head down, doodling on a serviette. Matt gripped his wife Janice's hand while she fiddled with his wedding ring. He had a deer-in-the-headlights look I knew well. Matt hated arguments and if this one heated up it would be close to the bone. Janice was the best example we knew of how ravaged a daughter could become by over-involvement.

Then Nancy spoke up. She knew all about co-dependence, she said. It happened to the adult children of alcoholics. So she knew about it in relation to drunks. But co-dependence with aging parents? That was a new one on her. I glared at Nancy, my jaw grinding. Did we need this red herring of alcoholism now? For years Nancy and I had argued about what was going on in the nightly cocktail hour of our childhood memories. She saw Mom and Dad as boozers. I saw them as fifties people with highballs a way of life. But Nancy had studied the matter more than I had, I did admit. Children were affected by their early observations and experiences. Nancy glanced back, seeing my mouthed, "Shut up," and mouthing back, "No!"

"Actually," she added calmly, "one of the ways that a psychiatrist identifies co-dependency is if no one is willing to talk about it."

"Busted!" I thought. We all started to chatter at once about Mom's proposal to move next door to Judi. We were a family that talked things out! Judi would take care of herself, she promised. Mom insisted that she didn't, and had never, and would never, turn her life over to Judi, or anyone else for that matter. She couldn't even imagine such a thing! I suppressed a giggle, or was it actually a sneer I was holding back? "Ya, right," I thought.

I felt rage engulf me. I knew the work it took to keep life going smoothly in Calgary. I directed my words to John. "You are dead right, John, about the daughters bearing the burdens of care. Judi is up to her neck in it. And I can tell you that none of us is doing enough to help her." Judi touched my arm in a warning. "Not now," she whispered. "Zip it!" But I was on a roll. "And you...sons? You go on with your lives as if nothing was different, and call yourselves the healthy ones? That's just bullshit!" I felt a flood of relief. I'd said it!

Mom cringed. Nancy smiled. John stared. Matt studied his hands. Chris looked at his watch. Judi was the peacemaker again: "Let's just agree to disagree on the whole co-dependence thing, John." We all sipped our coffee. "Burnout isn't pretty. But isn't there another angle to this whole caring-for-parents thing? I see it differently."

Now Judi was more eloquent than I had ever heard her. Her voice strong, she insisted she accepted the challenges of being the Daughter on Deck, welcomed them, in fact. It was about her striving for a purpose-filled life. Caregiving was something she believed in. Sure, we sibs were on the hook for helping with our parents' needs, too. Mom and Dad could use all our special gifts. Matt who never failed to make them laugh. Chris so practical. John filling Mom's soul as he had from the day he was born. Steve visiting with his family once a year. Nancy ready to pitch in, too, but much more aware than Judi and me about putting her own mask on first, the airplane analogy for sensible selfishness. Judi looked intensely at John.

"Being there for Mom and Dad is my calling, John, like you are called to be a priest. I will do it the best way I know how." Their eyes locked, and John nodded. Judi and John had a special bond and understood this concept of a calling. The two were committed Catholics while the rest of us had given up on that long before. Judi lived a life of faith. "I believe I am called by God to do this." John looked at his hands, and whispered, "Then so be it." He looked up and smiled at Judi.

"Do what you think is best," he said. Judi had won her point.

So now Judi went to Mom and hugged her. "Welcome to Hull Estates," she said. "You will be happy there, and I'll always be there to help."

That ended the family meeting. There was nothing left to say. Chris reminded us we all had to check out of the hotel before 11:00. Mom beamed. We kissed each other on the cheek and hugged Mom and soon the room was empty. By the next month, Mom had moved in below Judi. Forty-nine steps, Judi said. A new routine began and for a while all was well. I knew our Parent Project journey had turned a corner.

4

Seize the Day

"One day, memories will be all I have."

Mom's offhand comments often made me shudder. Like saying she would be paralyzed. I asked her where that idea came from and she said she didn't know. It was just a feeling. "Anyway, there's some kind of tough time down the road, of that I'm sure."

Her expectation of the good life ending encouraged me to fill what vitality she had left with memories to sustain her in those bad times coming. Besides, I'd read more than once that the dying regretted more what they didn't do than what they did.

One of the few things my parents could agree on was travel. Both loved it, especially in their zoomer senior years with solo trips when they didn't have to drag their children along, or put up with each other. Those days were long over. Mom could barely get around with her back pain and she couldn't trust her bowels or her gorge to keep things in. Hers was not a travelling body. Dad was never sure where he was now, or what was going on. He recalled distant events with delight, but the more recent ones were fuzzy. His was not a travelling mind. What could I do, I wondered, to help them have one last very special travel experience? I yearned to see the light in their eyes again and I wanted it to be me putting it there.

When I asked Dad if he had any place he still wanted to go, he didn't hesitate. Though he had never smoked, he wanted a stogie from Cuba. That would be difficult. I needed accessible emergency care with an octogenarian father on board. Cuba was out of the question. "How about Mexico?" I countered. My husband, daughter Fiona and I were planning a trip in the spring. Would he and Martha like to join us?

"Oooooh, I love Mexico," Dad replied, instantly enthusiastic. There were interesting Mayan ruins, he said, churches covered with gold, and great music for free on the streets. "But we have to go Dutch," he warned, "and you might as well know it now, I'm not made of money!"

"I get it Dad," I smiled, "you are a budget kind of guy. We'll keep things cheap, just the way you like."

The following March, as the snow swirled in Calgary, we were off. Our taxi was already snug when we arrived at Dad and Martha's seniors' residence. My husband raised his eyebrows at Martha's huge suitcase and began his travel twitch. "We need two taxis," he said. Dad scoffed. His son-in-law was just being a fuddy-duddy. If we sat sideways with our backpacks on our laps and sucked in our stomachs, we would all fit fine. Fiona could sit on my lap. We were speeding down the highway when Ed said, "You do have your passports, Fred?"

"Of course I do!" Dad scoffed, patting his pockets to prove it.

"Well...can I see them?" Dad fumbled for a while, pulling dirty tissues and gum wrappers and old receipts out of every pocket and then rifling through his backpack.

"Must have forgotten them." Ed studied his watch, and muttered we didn't have time for this nonsense. I reached forward from the back seat to poke him, comfortable in the front, and glared at him in the rear view mirror. "Good thing we have to go back," Dad said cheerfully as the taxi U-turned. "I forgot all my research about Mexico."

"The meter is running, sir," the driver reminded us.

"Make it snappy," Ed barked.

Dad held my arm and we shuffled as fast as we could, but Dad couldn't move faster than a plod. Once inside, he went straight to his desk, and there the passports were, on top of a bundle of photocopies from the best parts of *Lonely Planet*, his research. What were those other papers on the desk, all saying 'Final Notice'? I made a mental note to talk to Judi about that. Another job was coming her way. We were off again. "Got your money?" Ed asked. I jabbed my husband, warning him not to push his luck with me. Petulant now, Dad waved his travelers cheques. "Satisfied?" They were in $10 denominations, for a total of $200, Canadian funds. This wouldn't go far in Mexico, for two people and two weeks, even going Dutch, I knew. But I kept my mouth shut and blessed Ed for his silence, too. Dad would have budgeted with great care, using his memory of two decades before of what things cost. And currency confused him.

"You have to take that off, sir." The security officer had spotted the bulky pouch around Dad's middle. "You can't go through Security wearing that." Dad was tired now. It made him testy in the way that always made me cringe. Before I could stop him, Dad had undone his belt and pulled down his pants to reveal the secret belt and well-worn shorts. The hidden pouch revealed dozens of batteries for his hearing aids, tiny tubes of

41

toothpaste, some Vaseline, and a skinny wad of emergency cash. Was that pill wrapped in Saran Wrap really Viagra?

"Do you want my pacemaker, too?" Dad was unbuttoning his shirt. "Pacemaker, sir? You have a pacemaker? You can't go through a scanner with that!" That meant Dad had to line up for a pat-down, while Ed studied his watch, his jaw clenched. We piled Dad and Martha into wheelchairs to sprint to the boarding gate with minutes to spare. All the way, Dad tried to tell me that he didn't mind having his scrotum squeezed.

"Forget it, Dad," I cut him off. "I don't want to know about your balls."

Dad wanted the window seat, but also warned me he needed to tinkle every half hour or so. I was happy to leave chatty Martha with Ed and Fiona. They had better skills for tuning out. Back and forth, back and forth, back and forth Dad and I shuffled to the washroom at the back. When he wasn't tinkling, Dad snored. I wondered how he could breathe with his head so pressed onto his chest. I was shocked, seeing him up close this way. Dad had been covering his physical infirmities at the same time as Martha had been revealing his mental ones at every opportunity.

In Mexican Customs, Martha hit the button that randomly determined who would be searched, and it flashed red. As the agents pulled her luggage apart, I marveled. She had an array of lingerie, a jug of shampoo big enough to keep a hair salon happy, and a range of outfits suitable for a honeymoon.

When we opened the door at the top of too many stairs and saw our budget room at Casa Maria, my heart skipped a beat. How could we manage in this dive for ten days? There was one big room, with room dividers waist high separating the beds, like a hostel. The toilet wheezed. Dad thought the place was charming. Though a terrace on the roof up a spiral metal staircase had a commanding view over the city, our window looked out on a brick wall. I vowed to make the best of things.

"Yes, Dad, this place is going to be just fine."

"Do you think Grandpa and Martha were—"

I wouldn't let Fiona finish. "Yes," I said, "they were. But let's not say anything." The grunts and wheezes the night before, coming from the scratchy bed springs that suggested Dad and Martha were not sleeping, had kept us all awake. "I'll get us earplugs."

Cramming five people into taxis was normal in Mexico. But Dad thought 30 pesos was highway robbery and said the bus would only cost us five. What spendthrifts we were! I ignored him. The taxi was two dollars.

We were eager to start sightseeing, and though Dad had worked out his top-ten list, he was exhausted and breathing heavily within minutes. All he really wanted to do was watch the world go by. Now Ed was twitching with impatience and Fiona looked uncomfortable as Martha harangued Dad to get a move on.

"Hey, Dad, why don't we just sit and enjoy the *zócalo*? I'd love to hang out with you. Let's let everyone else go exploring. We can just rest." That time was memorable. Dad and I sat on the ornate metal benches in the plaza, in the shade of sculpted laurel trees, and watched the mariachis, the vendors with their monster clouds of bright helium balloons, the children and the couples strolling around in their Sunday best. We didn't need to talk. It was fun just being together. Sheepishly, I reached to hold Dad's hand. That was a little too much for him, though. He pulled away.

Dinners were a challenge, especially when the bill came. "Remember, we are going Dutch," Dad would say each time, and pass Ed a twenty-peso note, worth a dollar and a half. He didn't have any idea about exchange rates, and twenty bucks was plenty to feed two people in a cheap place like Mexico. Without a word Ed filled in the several-hundred-peso gap and assured Dad he'd left a tip. Money didn't matter. We could get more. The important thing was Dad's pride that he was paying his way.

Inevitably, Montezuma's Revenge caught up to Dad. Washing hands was sissy, he said, and salad kept him regular. All night we endured his gassy shuffle, the flicking lights and the multiple flushes of the empty toilet tank. Ed whispered about a whiff of something awful and I told him to just go back to sleep. When we woke the next day, shredded grey underpants were draped over the chairs. Fiona wondered if buying some new briefs might be a solution to this problem, but Dad was snarky. "I have plenty of new ones at home," he snapped. "That's a waste of money." I felt sorry for my father and his lost dignity. Anything to do with bowels was shameful.

We spent our last few days at a beach. As the taxi sailed past the high-end resorts between the airport and the water, Martha started to complain. Why weren't we stopping at a hotel with a pool and a garden and air conditioning, she wondered. Dad gloated, though. We were coming to "the real Mexico," just like he remembered it. At the end of the road was a line of rustic one-room huts with thatched roofs and tiny verandas. The fans clacked and there were flyspecks on the mosquito nets and the taps groaned. Was this clutch of plastic tables and chairs sporting beer logos really the restaurant? Though this rarely happened, I agreed with Martha.

Casa de Los Suenos was a dump. But it was right on the beach, with clear green-blue water dotted with cruise ships looking out onto cloudless skies filled with flocks of pelicans. It was Dad's place of dreams.

Each morning after fried fish with our eggs and fresh pineapple, Fi and I hoisted Dad to his feet and held him securely by both arms as he waddled across the sand to the water's edge. He cooed as we inched him into the warm ocean for what he referred to as his dip. The threadbare and faded bathing suit reached up just under his nipples. His pacemaker bulged through his saggy skin with his lady breasts. The thatch of curly chest hair that always impressed me as a kid was now a woolly grey. Once up to his waist in the ocean, Dad swirled his arms and slapped the waves with the abandon of a child. He said the fish nipped his feet and the sand was squishy and it was fun. He was shivering in no time, though, so we helped him back to lie for a moment or two on the sand on his worn travelling towel. "I thought I would never use this gear again," he said each time we went through this swimming routine. Then, for the rest of each day, he lay in a hammock under the palms and read the same chapter of his bodice-ripper until he fell asleep. I took his arm each time he said he had a tinkle coming, and helped him to the toilet. Three days later the taxi came back for us, and dropped us back at the airport.

"What is this place called?" Dad asked again and again. Ed repeated the name, over and over, "Zee-what-in-eh-oh." Finally, he gave up. "Mexico, Fred, it's just Mexico."

"Oh, Mexico. Well, it's way better than Cuba," was Dad's reply. Things went downhill fast for Dad in the months after that. I never regretted seizing the day and taking him on that last trip of his life.

I asked Mom, on one of her visits to the Coast, if there was anything she wanted to see or do. We both knew it would have to be a simple adventure, and close by, too. Her back pain would not let her sit in a car for long. Mom wanted to visit the Pacific Rim, a town called Tofino. It looked out on nothing but eagles and seagulls, waves and fog, with no land all the way to Japan. I could rent a cabin looking out at the ocean. Mom said a maritime sojourn would be a dream come true for her.

I was worried. Travel with Mom was a risky venture. I packed everything I could think of, fearful that some forgotten item would turn a pleasant two days into a nightmare. I packed her special chair that was a cross between a garden lounger and the cockpit of a space capsule. It held Mom in an almost upside-down position called zero gravity. Nothing pressed on her back in this position, so it was comfortable. I packed extra blankets just in case, a hot water bottle, and a heating pad because Mom suffered from the cold. I packed more pills than she needed, and a mass of incontinence pads I hoped she would not need. I double-checked that there were enough big bottles of Diet Coke and a 40-ounce jug of rum.

And cartons of her Matinee cigarettes. That part worried me. The rented cabin had a view beyond compare, a Jacuzzi, fireplace and huge TV screen. But the rule was "Absolutely No Smoking." I rented it anyway. No place worth staying in allowed smoking any more. So I also packed cans of air freshener, incense and smoke-eating candles. If we got caught, I had cash to pay the fine. We would get caught, I was sure. Mom filled any room she occupied with clouds of acrid smog.

The drive left Mom sore and tired. She said all she wanted was a rum and a rest with a fire to warm her. The

46

wood was damp to the touch, but I had plenty of firelighters and got right to it. Proud of my Girl Guide wood arrangement, I didn't even check to be sure the chimney damper was open. It wasn't. As the wood began to burn, smoke began to fill the room. I jangled the hot metal draft lever, swearing and in panic, while Mom prayed, "Please God, if it be your will, make this problem go away." It did. "Amen," she said as the smoke began to rise up the chimney. She lit her first cigarette.

God heard my prayer, too. The pall from the fireplace made our eyes stream water and sting, but it overpowered any cigarette pong. "Bliss," Mom said, "you are such a good daughter."

For the next two days we played Scrabble and didn't call each other for cheating. We drank. We never turned off the TV. It triggered a memory for me of our days at the Millennium in Ottawa five years before. Like then, she told me stories. Like then, I asked her all the questions that came to my mind, to keep her talking. How was her time working in the House of the Dying in Calcutta? Did Mother Teresa deserve to be canonized as a saint? Mom told me how she loved living in Mother Teresa's convent and how she made friends with the street dwellers outside the walls and the rats that scattered under her bed sometimes. I asked her about her adventures in China. How did she communicate with Nadia, the Russian-speaking fellow teacher who spoke no English? How could they travel around China together on third-class trains? If their only common language was French and Mom knew no more than a hundred appallingly pronounced words, how could they have become such friends? Most of all, I wanted to know about Mom's flight to the desert island off the coast of Belize. Why did she feel she must escape from

Dad? Even more curious to me, why did she feel she must drag my little brothers on the lam with her that time? The thought of how unfair that was to everyone still made me angry after all these years. She said she had grown tired of trailing after Dad in his career at the cost to her own. She was tired, she said, of putting herself second. The six-month contract teaching in the one-room school and being the only nurse on the Belizean island had seemed too good to pass up. She remembered fondly how she and her two little boys played Swiss Family Robinson, eating fish and fruit and slapping sand flies and sleeping in the sea breezes on their hammocks. "I never regretted it," she said, "but now I want a nap."

Mom was popping an awful lot of pills. She didn't know what they were for exactly, saying she trusted her doctor and friend, Nan, to give her what she needed. I wasn't so sure. Judi and I called Dr. Nan Mom's pusher. Every time Judi took Mom to an appointment they left with another prescription for some new drug to overcome the effects of something else. Mom gobbled them in handfuls with a swig of rum to wash them down. Was she addicted to some of them? This wasn't a time to challenge her. I made a note to talk to Judi about it. We watched the sun go down and the moon rise and the stars dance on the waves glowing with bioluminescence. I read to her. When she napped I went out to breathe fresh ocean air and buy fat crab from the fishermen on the dock. She smacked her lips as we ate off newspaper and didn't care as butter dribbled down our chins.

One thing was missing, though. How could I get Mom right to the ocean's edge? She said she wanted to wet her toes in the Wild Pacific. Long Beach had a wide expanse of loose sand, too difficult for Mom to navigate. I got the miracle I needed. It came in the form of a small poster outside the bakery where I'd bought sourdough bread to go with the crab. "Beach Wheelchair on loan. National Park Visitors Centre." I smiled. All Canadians had a right to dip their toes in the Pacific, no matter how crocked up they were.

Mom was thrilled but anxious as the ranger loaded her into the specially designed dune buggy and tipped it way back. I tucked a blanket around her and we were off. The path to the water's edge threaded through driftwood logs that people had made into lean-tos and sculptures. Then we glided along hard sand for almost a mile, as Mom pointed out the bull kelp and the blobs of jellyfish and the shells, squealing with delight at the smell of the sea. Eagles soared above and the waves lapped, now at her feet when we stopped for a while. Finally, the tide began to turn and a foghorn signaled rain on the way. It was suddenly cool. Mom said her back was hurting.

When we got back to the car I passed Mom her pain pills and she took double the recommended dose. I looked the other way. Then I tucked her onto the back seat of the car, propped pillows just so under her neck and knees, and covered her with a blanket. She was asleep in minutes. She didn't budge until I pulled into my driveway. Had she overdosed? I kept looking over my shoulder at her as I drove, hoping that she was OK.

She was. "You are such a worry wart," Mom said. "Can't a lady have a nap?" There was no place like home, I said as I passed her a tall glass of rum and Coke. Mom didn't completely agree about that. Sure, home was more comfortable. But being a lump on a log didn't make memories the way travel did. Her extra dose of pain was worth it. "We'll do this again," I assured her, and she said, "Soon," and we both knew we were lying. It was one of those comfortable fibs, though, the kind that kept us focused on the bright side, where there was hope and life left to be lived.

Mom said again what she so often said these days: "One day, memories will be all I have."

How could she know that? "Don't say that, Mom." I was gloomy when she was pessimistic about what lay ahead.

"No sense pretending," she said. "It is what it is."

5

Pretending

"If I pretend to be fine, I will be fine."

In the space of a week, Mom morphed from sports indifference to an obsession with hockey. The home team was doing well and Mom caught the excitement of the race to the Stanley Cup. The Flames were on fire, and so was she. I was visiting Calgary to cover for Judi on an upcoming trip she was taking with her husband. As usual I arrived a few days earlier for twin time. We drove home from the airport with Flames flags flapping from the window of the car. Now we were in Mom's living room to watch the big game on TV. She wore a red T-shirt with the team crest and the name Kiprusoff on the back. This was the goalie, she explained, and her favorite player. The Kip reminded her of Matt. She also wore her Lady Diana wig, the one she saved for the times she was feeling really sparky. I loved the energy this wig seemed to deliver, like some magic. The pretend hairdo meant real celebration.

The third period was ending and the win was secure. Cowbells were clanging on the Red Mile just two blocks away. That was the street where Calgarians swarmed after a hockey game. Mom wanted to get there to feel the excitement firsthand. We were missing out, she badgered. "What are we waiting for?"

Judi and I shared a glance – was Mom getting manic? I shrugged. So often, the upswing of her mood was followed by a slump. Was it going to be a problem this time? There was no doubt. Mom seemed to be having more fun than she'd had in a long time. Manic or not, I loved this zip that Mom produced only rarely now. "Come on girls! Let's just get a wiggle on!"

Getting to the Red Mile was going to be a challenge. Mom could not walk two blocks. Some weeks before, her back had begun to pound with spiking pains, making every step a form of torture. No one could say why that was or if it would get better or worse, but Dr. Nan offered more pain medications, as she always did. Two weeks before, there had been a crisis when Mom could not even walk the hall from her car in the garage to the elevator, and then the long hall back to her apartment on the 14th floor. As always, Judi came to the rescue, and pushed Mom back to the comfort of her recliner in a jerry-rigged wheelchair, an office chair on tiny wheels. Since then, both of them were afraid to try another excursion. Walk to the Red Mile? Impossible!

The horn sounded the end of the game and the Flames were on their way to the final. Cheers rose to a crescendo from the street. Mom pleaded again, "Let's just go!"

It was time to bring up the topic of the wheelchair again. Judi had bought it the day after the office-chair rescue. Mom refused to look at it. "If I sit in that thing once, I'll never get out of it. I don't want that. Can't you understand?" I did understand. Mom wasn't ready to see herself as crippled. So the wheelchair remained shrouded in plastic, hidden in the back of Mom's cupboard behind her winter coats. On the subject of moving around, we were in an impasse.

"You will have to ride in the wheelchair," Judi said. She could be as stubborn as Mom. "You can't walk. I want to go to the Red Mile. I want to take you. But I'm not taking you any other way." Mom glared. There was a heavy silence in the apartment that only made the sounds of cheering on the Red Mile more enticing. Finally, Mom gave in. "OK you win, I will ride just this once, just to make you happy."

"We are happy," I grinned. "Let's get a move on."

We struggled with the unfamiliar contraption, while Mom sat in her La-Z-Boy, smoking and offering advice. How did it unfold? How did the footsies attach? How did the brake work? Finally, we were ready and Mom settled into the seat, muttering that this was not a good idea but let's get going, and we were off on our maiden voyage.

Mom might be right, I thought, but too bad. She needed to stop pretending that she was more whole than the reality of her crumbled back. Perhaps we were turning a caregiving corner, toward loss of mobility, but too bad! The wheelchair meant more freedom for everyone. Like it or not, it had to be. What better motivation to accept the inevitable than the fun happening on the Red Mile?

The curbs were the hardest part. Judi stomped on the bar on the back of the chair and tipped it, while I gripped the arms to keep the chair from toppling sideways. Mom keened in terror, "Don't drop me, I know I am going to fall!" But between these obstacles, she waved her arms in the Flames victory salute yelling, "Go team go!" Passersby smiled benignly at this excited old fan. Over the buildings we could see the tip of the white roof of the hockey arena, shaped like a saddle and glowing with its interior lights. Beside it were the blazing lights of the Stampede race track.

"Remember how we went to the races, Mom?" I was feeling nostalgic. It had been years since we walked together that Saturday afternoon during one of my visits to Calgary. I reminded her how she put a dollar in her pocket to give to the first panhandler and then pretend to be out of money when the next one asked for spare change. It was a lie. She had a pocket full of money for betting, but in another way it was a fact: none of her change after that giveaway dollar coin was spare. At the track, Mom explained her power of positive thinking strategy of betting. First she went to the wagering window and placed her orange $2 bill on the horse with the worst odds. Then she kissed her ticket for luck and we hustled to the paddock where the horses were being paraded. When Mom saw her horse she shouted with a frenzy of encouragement, "Way to go!" The jockey looked around at probably the only fan who believed in him. "If I pretend he's going to win, maybe he will." That never happened, but it wasn't the point. Mom wanted her support to be a morale boost for the jockey, win or lose. I smiled when I remembered. That day with Mom was not so long ago, and then she could walk faster than I could.

Now we were on the Red Mile. Drunks surged around the wheelchair and Mom complained she couldn't see anything except asses. She shouted "Go Flames Go" a few times, but Judi and I could see how her face had morphed from giddy to grave. "Want a hot dog?" I asked. Mom clutched her stomach but wanly agreed. She could only manage a nibble off the corner before she passed it to me. "I can't eat it. My stomach is turning. I need to get to the bathroom. I need to get home. Can we go now? Fast?"

"Let me get a picture at least." Judi fiddled with the camera. "This is a historic occasion after all." She snapped a quick pose of Mom seeming to wave the hot dog in the air. Then, we headed for the barn like range ponies smelling hay. Mom clutched her stomach and moaned. Judi jumped the curbs as we careened along. I went ahead asking celebrating drunks to make way for a wheelchair. It was nip and tuck. Mom made it to the bathroom just before she erupted at both ends.

If the adventure was not a winner, the picture of the adventure was. Mom looked spectacular, and she knew it. "I actually look happy, don't I?" she said. "I don't feel that way very often these days." I suggested that we send the picture of Mom looking so well to 'the list'. This was the email group of twenty or more family members and friends whom Judi kept informed of the slow-motion fade of Mom and Dad. Both Judi and I were committed to communication with our siblings. They weren't able to help much, but still said they wanted to have news. We felt it was part of the Parent Project to keep everyone up to speed. And there hadn't been much good news to share for a while. An upbeat vignette of the Red Mile, less the explosions at the end, was overdue.

The reactions to the picture came quickly. Steve's was first. He was so pleased to see Mom looking so good, he began. But he wondered if we had we been over-reacting to her troubles before, maybe even exaggerating? Chris suspected the same thing in his straight-shooter way. "I'm confused. What is really going on with Mom? Can you make up your minds about how she is doing?" Nancy said she was relieved that things seemed to be picking up for Mom. Could she put off that planned trip to help out? Things were awfully busy in her life these days. If Mom was fine, coming for a visit in a few more months would work better in her schedule. John wondered if Mom was manipulating us. Was she presenting herself as feeling terrible when scratch the surface and she was just the opposite? Matt said he wished he'd been there for a bite of the hot dog. Great, he added, that Mom was back to her old self.

All these reactions left me unsettled. Was John right that Mom was faking her condition to manipulate? Were we caught in her web of pretended incapacity, or even spinning lies of our own? Were Chris and Steve right to be annoyed that we kept changing the story? What was true? Did we have some subconscious need for Mom and Dad to be feeble? Did they have an agenda to get more attention than they really needed? That was one of the tough parts of the Parent Project. We were never certain what was too little or too much. Was it a disservice to Mom to respond to her as not being well? Was our response a self-fulfilling prophecy? Was Mom relieved to know we understood her, grateful for her good daughters? Or, was she descending to our low expectations? No, I told myself, we were supporting her, in this dance of care and being cared for, accepting all the ups and downs for what they were without judgment. But it was complicated. Judi was just furious. How dare these siblings to second-guess our understanding of how things are from their freedom of the peanut gallery! Let them come and try to do better!

The word storm passed. Mom liked having this picture to remind her she still had the ability to be fun-loving sometimes. She said she was glad that it had triggered responses from her children, whether or not we twins were happy with them. And for heaven's sake, she added, she was like anyone else in the world. Some days were good days. Others rotten. What was the matter with putting on her best face, anyway?

I was left with a new residue of uncertainty about our caregiving. Did our thinking make it so, just as Hamlet said? Did treating Mom as an invalid make her into one? What about the wheelchair? Was it really a good idea?

In the end I decided to go with Mom's conclusion from the aborted adventure on the Red Mile. "If I pretend that I am fine," she said, "I will be fine." That was not so hard to accept, was it?

6

Finding Meaning

"You are such a good daughter."

Both Mom and Dad got a kick out of volunteering. They said they liked the kind of people they met when they were helping out. They felt happy to think that their efforts moved the dial even a smidgen to make a better world. In my childhood, Mom and Dad seemed to like each other best when they were volunteering together.

I used to sit on the stairs in my pre-teen years, out of sight but watching Mom and Dad having fun every Tuesday with the club they had set up to send ten thousand books to a school library in India. Five couples filled the living room those nights. There was laughing and talking and even some singing as they knelt on the floor wrestling bundles of old texts. Some cut the stiff paper to size. Getting the string tight around the wrapping was a job for two. Someone else did the inky job of addressing the packages. When the books were packed and a pile of bundles sat by the door, it was time to relax over coffee and date squares or banana bread. Once a month I went with Dad to the post office to send the packages on their way by sea mail. On many Saturdays I entertained my little brothers while Mom baked pies to sell at bazaars and Dad collected beer bottles with his cronies, all to earn the postage money. The image of this commitment was my template for dedication to a higher cause.

Years later, now almost twenty and a University graduate with no firm direction yet, I volunteered in the same school in India. My task was to sort and catalogue the books for the library and finally, after years, get them on the shelves. My shock was profound when I saw them. The thousands of bundles were still unwrapped. They were stacked floor to ceiling in a dingy storeroom, greenish and smelling of mold. Eventually, they all had to be burned, in a bonfire of broken dreams. I was appalled that the years of work in my childhood living room proved to be fruitless. The project did not reach its goal. This was a weight on my mind and a barrier between me and my parents, like any secrets are. Decades later, in some conversation now forgotten, I released myself of the burden by telling her this story. I explained that I'd kept the secret for so many years because I didn't want to hurt her and Dad, knowing how great that effort had been. "That's OK." Mom smoked a few moments before she said more. The goal was only part of the whole project, not even the most important part. The process was what really mattered to her. The only thing she could control was her bit, and she knew she had done it well. The pile of ash? "Well," she said, patting my hand, "everything happens for a reason you know, and for all I know that library of Canadian books might have been a bad idea. So it doesn't matter to me." Of all Mom's life lessons, this was wisdom that stuck. Forget how it ends. That's not in your hands. Focus on the process. That's what really matters. As a caregiver, staying in the present moment often saved me from despair.

Now, as the first decade of the millennium reached its mid-point, and my parents dwindled more each month, they still found ways to give back. For Dad, it was pop cans. When he found out that each empty can fetched three cents at the nearby recycle depot, he was hooked into the subculture of the bottle people. Other bored old men in Dad's seniors' residence thought can and bottle collecting would be fun, too, so a group began scrounging the garbage for a mystery cause. I asked Dad once if he knew how the money was to be used. "Nope," he said, "that's not my job." He seemed bemused that I would want to know a detail like that.

Though he staggered now, Dad still got out every day. He called the local recreation centre his spa and never missed his swim and can-collecting routine. Going and coming, he stuck his head in every garbage bin. Once a passing driver saw this and called the police, concerned an old man had wandered away from the nearby Alzheimer Care Centre. The driver described Dad with his beaten up safari hat and nylon backpack, bulging and in shreds. The officer thanked the Good Samaritan and said the old geezer was well known to the detachment, and he was fine.

The lifeguards cheered for Dad as he flashed his pass and toothy false teeth grin. They said he was a model to all the kids of a never-give-up old guy who stayed active even when he could barely walk. They kept a close eye on him, though, as he wheezed through five widths of the pool and had a nap on the plastic lounge chairs in the sunshine before heading home, still hunting for treasure. Three hundred cans earned $9! But the really big money was in pull tops. He had twist-top sandwich bags full of these aluminum tabs, and no present gave Dad more pleasure than a fistful to add to his collection. Even at the end of his life, when he couldn't get out of his chair and wasn't sure where he was, Dad's face lit up when a pull tab came his way. If the meaning of life was the journey, Dad was on a joy ride.

Mom's search for meaning was way more complex than Dad's. She wanted to stretch her mind, or change her perspective, and she wanted to be meeting interesting people. That's why mentoring was Mom's perfect volunteer activity as she slowed down. She had plenty to share and no one could listen as intently as Mom for what was said and left unsaid. I found Adele's plea for work as a geriatric massage therapist buried under other job-seeker cards on a hospital notice board. Since Mom was always sore somewhere, Adele's offerings seemed worth trying. I knew that Mom would refuse to spend what she would call a king's ransom to hire Adele, so I did. "Happy Birthday, Mom!" I told her, "and your present is ..." Put that way, Mom accepted three months of weekly massages to see if they were helpful for pain reduction but also a pleasant experience, both my important criteria for my gift. Little did I know that Adele would give much more than a massage.

The two women hit it off on many levels. She was a graduate of one of the programs that was developed under Mom's tenure in the corner office. Sampling the product of her earlier intelligence was one thing, but Mom loved even more to offer guidance to Adele about the secret wishes of old ladies for touch. Who knew? Mom said she missed the sensations of being stroked in a loving way. So Adele ran her fingers through Mom's hair as well as gently massaging the tight spots all over Mom's body. It was exquisite pleasure, Mom said.

They talked nonstop while Adele rubbed. What was it like to be really old? What were the trials of being a single mom? How could Adele's business be expanded and built to meet her deep desire to make a significant difference for the elderly using the talent in her gentle hands? And how was Adele's mother doing as she shriveled in a long-term-care centre under the onslaught of Alzheimer's? What books were they reading? What was on TV? Judi and I guessed that we were topics of conversation, too. We were more than OK with that. It was release. And Adele, a caregiver to her mother, knew where we were coming from as caregivers. Long after the birthday present was over, Mom kept on with Adele visits every week, and paid her more than well. Adele needed that steady infusion of cash. Business with the very old could be spotty. The two became inseparable parts of each other's success in beating what were their different challenges, being old and serving the elderly. It was mutual mentoring.

Mom also met weekly with nursing students. Every Monday afternoon through three semesters, a half dozen young women knocked on Mom's door. Tea was ready, thanks to Judi. For a couple of hours, they listened as Mom told her stories of being a wartime nurse, or being the only medical person on a desert island in the Caribbean, or what it was like helping the dying picked up off the streets of Calcutta. She told them how wounds were treated in the days before antibiotics, and broken bones set. She had plenty of advice about child-rearing for the two nursing students who were also moms. She listened as they talked about the demands placed on them as learners in that long-ago training kingdom where she reigned. It was a two-way street of sharing and Mom loved the experience. Alas, it ended. The program changed and the next batch of students would go to push juice carts or whatever odd jobs would put them in an Alzheimer's care centre. I followed up and learned that the powers that be were disappointed with Mom as mentor. They wanted their students to experience cognitive frailty. Mom was certainly not delivering that result. Everyone lost, I thought, when the mentoring was over. It had given Mom joy to share her experience. I believed she had made a difference.

The end of the student mentoring was not the end of mentoring, though. It happened again in a different way. Word had travelled to a filmmaker about Mom and her caregiving twin daughters. He was preparing a series of six documentaries titled, *Aging in the Modern World*. It would explore aspects and issues of aging that were never discussed in textbooks. The series would support a program training nurses specializing in geriatrics. Mom was a rare find. There were not many seniors as old and as infirm as she was, still willing and able to participate in a filming schedule that might be grueling and would certainly have tight timelines. Not only that, he'd heard that she was witty, thoughtful and articulate, and Judi and I were interesting, too. Together we were just what the film-maker was looking for, Judi reported. Daughter on Deck and Daughter at a Distance, we both said in the same breath, as if we rehearsed. Then we laughed, excited about the prospect of telling our story from all sorts of angles.

Judi had one more reason than me to be thrilled. This film-maker was a mover and shaker in communications, her field, and he just might help her inject new juice into her dehydrated career. She hated being a has-been. And me? I always looked forward to twin time, especially the kind where Judi was not packing her bags to travel to someplace exotic with her husband, Tom, the day after I arrived in Calgary to cover for her. But there was more in this for both of us. Perhaps we would all be prodded to dig more deeply into the Parent Project, not skim its surface, as we just did the work with little reflection. Preparing for being filmed, we might be able to talk about the bigger picture things that viewers might like to hear, and I certainly did. I wanted to know from Mom and Judi about their best times and worst times in caregiving and being cared for, and what made them be that way? What did Mom still want to accomplish or learn as her life was winding down in slow motion? Did she fear death? Most of all, why did she use the phrase 'such a good daughter'? Judi agreed with me. She was curious, too. We could use the time of waiting for filming to get started to dig into some deeper conversations.

Mom was intrigued but anxious. Would there be too many demands? What if she wasn't feeling well when the filming was supposed to happen? Could she pull out at the last minute? Would she be able to say no to questions that she didn't feel like answering? I assured her every time a new worry popped up that we would handle everything and it would all be A-OK. It was all a fib. There would be tight schedules and tough questions and she would not be able to just pull out at the last minute. But I hoped Judi and I could manage Mom and her fears when the time arrived.

There were two elements to our part of the documentary. In the first, a film crew came into Mom's apartment and talked to us individually. Then we talked together. In the second element, a film crew followed us around with cameras and lights and dollies and microphones on long poles. That part was called B-roll. We looked forward to this adventure.

Two weeks before the filming date, Mom was manic. Her mind was spinning with ideas she wanted to share. Would I help her throw an opening party? When was I coming to

Calgary? She couldn't wait to see me. Perhaps we could practice? Judi and I began to worry. After manic, came depressed. On cue, that is what happened. Judi knocked on Mom's door for her morning check-in and did not hear the faint but cheerful, "Come in, dear!" She found Mom sitting in the dark, her curtains drawn, the TV off. Mom told her to go away, and cancel the damn movie.

Judi was angry on the phone. "Every plan I make winds up this way, she's just so bloody irritating when she gets like that!" I soothed her and said Mom had a medical issue, she was not being ornery on purpose. I changed my flight plans to arrive earlier in Calgary than I had planned. Judi needed backup in this sticky situation, and usually my arrival jollied Mom out of her funks. My plan was to focus her on how this film was mentoring and how mentoring was her gift to the universe. She needed that perspective. Just in case, I called the producer to say Mom wasn't well and the crew might need to reschedule.

"Hi Mom, it's me, Janet, can I come in?" This was the moment of truth.

"Of course you can, dear!" Relief! The mood had shifted again. She was back to her bubbly self. She said she was counting the days until filming and hoped Judi had not taken her seriously saying she wanted to cancel it. Of course she wanted to be part of *Aging in the Modern World*. Her curtains were open, the lights were on and the best sign of all, CNN was back blaring on the TV. Yes, all was well, she assured me. "Why don't you brew a pot of coffee and we can brainstorm about what questions might be asked?"

The film crew dragged an astounding amount of gear into Mom's apartment. There were lights on stands and many microphones, blackout curtains and silver reflectors to be propped at every angle. A crowd filled the living room. There was the producer, the director, and an interviewer. There was a camera operator and sound technician and even a woman fixing us up with powder and brushes and rouge. She clipped our clothes to look right and threaded microphones through our sleeves.

Mom went first.

"Roll 'em," the director said. "May I call you Betty?" the interviewer asked with a smile. Mom flashed a demure look. "Yes, you may." She relaxed then. People who asked her how she wanted to be addressed went in her good books in that instant. It was respectful, she said. For the next hour he worked through his questions, following Mom's lead through a conversation about the inner work of aging. I realized how much Mom's early experiences had made her stoical and sometimes secretive. Her toddler trauma with the broken glass might have set her on the path of endurance without complaint, when complaint was an appropriate response. Caring for her grandmother and mother might have formed her ideas about what good care was all about, and made her fearful now. And being a spy? Of course Mom was hardwired to keep things to herself while getting everyone else to talk. I could see now how her beliefs about life helped and hindered her now that she was coming to its edge.

Mom wanted most of all to tell the interviewer how being Catholic was making her old age easier. The interviewer was skillful, and redirected this so that she was not talking about a particular set of religious beliefs, but sharing her understanding of how she saw suffering as part of life. Mom would have none of that. Endurance in suffering, "offering it up" in this life, would reduce her sentence for sins committed in the next. That was how the Catholics saw it. She might get out of purgatory and on to heaven quicker, she explained, having done her time in purgatory while still on earth. As Mom went on, parrying with the interviewer, I began to be concerned. Some of this felt too quirky to me. *Aging in the Modern World* was not destined for the Vision Channel, after all! When she started to talk about how she used ejaculations in prayer, though, I prickled with sweat.

"Cut!" The director and interviewer whispered among themselves while the make-up woman added a little more powder to Mom's forehead. Did they think she was getting batty? The camera rolled again. Perhaps they agreed in their huddle that Mom should just be free to talk, and they would be free afterwards to edit. The director smiled, though, when her sound bite came. "My spirituality sustains me," she said. "It is as simple as that." Viewers would all relate, whatever their beliefs. Some creed that placed life into a bigger picture was helpful at this end of life. I knew that sequence would make it to the final product.

"What kind of care do you need at this stage of your life?" Judi and I leaned forward, tense. This was about us. "Not much," Mom smiled. "I actually get around very well, though I do have a number of little problems here and there." I could feel more than hear Judi's teeth grind. Mom listed them. She had a heart condition, diabetes, spinal stenosis, macular degeneration, skin cancer, lung cancer, arthritis, fatigue, constant nausea, and sleep problems. Oh, yes, her bowels were beastly, too. "Other than that, I am fine." I knew Mom believed she was basically healthy. It was her world view. She saw her glass in life as half full and holding its own, not half empty and draining. She was grateful for her well-being, such as it was, and knew that health was a gift. That will be in the final product, too, I thought.

The interviewer turned to Mom's thoughts on death and dying. My stomach clenched. The death part was no problem, she explained, but dying made her uncomfortable when she allowed herself to contemplate it. She admitted that she was stuck in a vortex of losses and admitted she was losing patience, but she still loved life. I jabbed Judi. "Long Time Dying," I whispered, "sounds like a good title for a country song." She frowned and put her finger to her lips. Shhhh. This was no time for a joke.

"Do you want to hear about the time I died?" Mom asked. The interviewer raised his eyebrows a fraction, and glanced at the director. Was this old dame taking over the interview? Should he let her?

"Cut!" There was another huddle. I figured they were deciding if *Aging in the Modern World* would benefit by a near-death experience account. Lots of people were talking about that sort of thing now. So why not? This Betty Perry was coming on as a vivid storyteller. The vignette could be edited if necessary. The two men smiled and I knew they were ready to listen to what Mom was prepared to share.

"Roll the cameras," the director called.

"I do want to hear about your near-death experience." The interviewer leaned in, "Tell me, Betty. Tell me all about it in your own words." Mom smiled, slightly coy, I thought. This was by far her favorite story. To me it was a bizarre tale that left me feeling queasy when she told it after a rum or two.

"Accept her reality," I admonished myself. "She owns her story. But on national television?"

"Pay attention," Judi hissed.

It happened when Matt was born. Her labour went on for days and, by the end, she was in crisis. Her pelvic floor had ripped badly when Matt's head emerged and with his body came Mom's insides. She said she was not conscious, of course, but she was aware of everything happening below as the doctor worked to save her life and Matt's, too. As a watcher, she looked down from the lights on the chaos surrounding her. She heard the orders shouted, the hums of machines, the expletives. She saw the doctor stuffing her bowel inside her, basting her back together, and didn't care. The electric paddles came out and shocked her. She felt that at a distance but still didn't care. Mom cared most about the tunnel of light coming towards her. She was not afraid of it. She felt drawn in, and her whole being was suffused with joy and peace. "I felt the presence of everyone I loved who'd died before me, and they were all beckoning me to come to them." Now there was silence in Mom's apartment as everyone strained to hear. Mom said nothing for a few moments, too. We waited.

"And?" The interviewer probed in a whisper.

Mom said she couldn't describe the feeling. But she had a growing certainty that she must not follow that light. That baby needed her. She still had all those kids. Pulling back into her body and to her life as wife and mother was the hardest decision, she explained, she ever had to make. But it was also an easy one. "I just knew it was not my time."

Judi was unhappy with her interview. The director asked a surprise question, "Why do you do this?" Her answer left her feeling ruffled. She was confused about it, she confided to me later. But to the interviewer, Judi insisted that she didn't feel at all like a slave to this unasked-for job of caregiver. She acknowledged challenges balancing her needs as a mother herself, a grandmother and a wife. She had to let friends go, her fitness plans had been derailed and now she felt like a blimp. She was losing her competitive edge in her tough career and now contracts were thin. Money was a concern. She was not saving for her own retirement any more. But then, Judi repeated, she felt more satisfaction than loss in being Daughter on Deck. "Liar," I thought. "She sure has plenty of frustration when we talk about it." But as I listened, I began to understand. Judi did have two minds, and both held a part of her truth. Afterward Judi asked me if she'd done OK, did she sound intelligent, or did she come off as a whiner? I assured her that she was great. I admired her honesty, including her ambivalence, and said that was the most important part of her family caregiver's perspective on aging. I said what I liked the best was how she said her relationships with Mom and Dad were getting deeper in an adult-to-adult way, the more she was involved in their care.

"You never told me that before," I said.

"You never asked," she replied. "Maybe I didn't see it that way until I was poked to think more deeply about my gains and losses." I realized that was true. Our caregiving relationship was stuck on the day-to-day challenges, the costs, of the Parent Project more than its benefits. I made a note to focus more on the up sides the next time we fell into one of our booze-fuelled yaks we called "whine and cheesed." It would be better for both of us to keep our eyes on the big picture.

I couldn't add much when it was my turn. I had a bit part. A thousand miles and a time zone kept me out of the same day-to-day action of Daughter on Deck. Still, I talked about how I was helping in the role of Daughter at a Distance. I always took over in Calgary when Judi had to travel. I called those trips respite. I said it was harder for Mom and Dad to visit me on the Coast but now I went with them as a companion on the flights. They loved my house by the forest, set up for all their needs. There were electric recliners in all the places they might sit. There were grab bars and bath chairs and commodes. When they visited, I became a full-time caregiver and set aside my own interests for that time to focus on theirs. Time was my biggest gift to them, I figured.

There were other things. I researched every new symptom, condition and drug and passed the information back to Judi. Maybe some doctors found it annoying to be faced with Dr. Google, but I knew it empowered Judi. She could speak to the specialists with more authority and keep an eye open for new problems emerging.

I explained that my biggest support was psychological. "Judi's never alone with the job. She can present herself to the world as the eternal optimist, but bellyache to me." We spoke every day, I explained, and talked about everything without filters. Most days, we connected several times. We worked out problems together.

Mom thought the B-roll part of the movie-making was more fun than the talking part. She liked the hoopla. The crew followed her to the hot water pool where she walked around, pushing a pool noodle with Adele holding her arm as they chatted, getting exercise without pain. They followed her to the grocery store, where Judi ran around finding the things on her list, while Mom rested on her walker at the end of each aisle. There was a sequence of her feeling tomatoes for ripeness. The most fun was the crew at the airport, with Mom and me on our way to the Coast. The microphone hung over my head as I asked the agent for the special chair to get Mom right to her seat on the plane. I imagined there would be a call after we were boarded from the Calgary agent to alert the one at the other end that movie stars were on the plane. The B-roll was intended to support the series theme that frailty need not be the end of a productive life. I hoped it would be obvious to the viewers, as it was to Judi and me, that nothing in this productive life happened without lots of support.

A few months later, we had a family viewing of the final product. Judi brought the series of DVDs and the pizza and Mom sat in her recliner. We binge-watched through the whole six hours. Clever editing had made Mom an archetype of the long-suffering elder with many complex and chronic problems, still living a rich life. She was the contented dwindler and wise woman. Judi was the caregiver sandwiched between her children and her job. The subtlety of how crucial she was to Mom's quality of life didn't come out as well as I hoped, but her saintliness shone through. As the distant family member, I gave an impression of offering egregious advice. That portrayal made me cringe. I must talk to Judi about it some time, I thought. The three of us together told a vivid story, though. We agreed after it was over that it missed some shades of grey that were the truth beneath the truth. There was the ambiguity of caregiving for a parent in declining health. There was the mix of frustration and love in the same sentence sometimes. The fact of no end in sight was huge for me, and missed in the edit. Nor did the series capture how our love and gratitude for each other was growing along with Mom's vulnerability. The balance between caregiving and care receiving was the special sauce of our recipe for the Parent Project. If the series was designed for training, wasn't this the most critical bit? When it was over, there seemed little we could say.

"You looked great in your wig, Mom."

"They sure played up the twin theme."

"I looked fat."

Someone told Judi, years later, that the documentary was still being used in training of nurse's aides. A friend phoned me on the Coast, reporting with excitement that she saw me on the Learning Channel. I concluded that *Aging in the Modern World* was making some kind of difference. That was enough for me, though I never watched the series again.

7

Getting Help

"I need you."

M om tackled her goal of being a university graduate the way she did everything else she wanted in life, with gusto. At the same time, I was flirting with flunking out of university in second year. I felt like a failure by the age of eighteen. We were guaranteed to clash in those days. I needed freedom. She needed help. I was frustrated and rebellious. She was menopausal and psychotic.

Shame and threat were my mother's tools in those days to get me to do her bidding. I had to look after my little brothers while she studied, because there was no money for babysitters. I needed to keep the house spotless because we had to keep our student boarders happy. They paid a lot of the family bills, including the ones I ran up. Her stomach needed time to heal from the incisions that had removed everything female, so there was no way she could push a vacuum or scrub a floor. Or carry heavy objects. That was the worst. Mom needed me to carry her books around campus. I was sometimes faint with fury. I had this role because I was the only child who could. My sisters had escaped. Judi because she couldn't stand Mom, both of them with unruly hormones, and Nancy because she felt Mom couldn't stand her.

My worst nightmare unfolded when Mom signed up for the same class I was taking, the one I called "No Fear Shakespeare." Mom called it "My dream come true." I said I would go on strike if she barged into my student life this way. No babysitting, no sheet washing, no toilet scrubbing. Mom tried flattery to get my cooperation. I was just so much smarter about writing essays and taking notes than she was. I knew how the library worked and she didn't. I just knew the score. Never! I remained adamant. Then she tried to lure me with promises of making my life easier. We could study together. She could give me her thoughts on Shakespeare. I recoiled. No way! Mom tried shame. What right did I have to tell her what classes she could take? I said I had no right but I was doing it anyway. Tough luck! Finally, she hit the jackpot with guilt. She thought I was a better daughter than apparently I turned out to be. "OK," I said. "Just this class. Just this once, damn it!"

I shriveled in embarrassment as my mother and I edged into the crowded classroom on the first day, me tagging along behind her and carrying the heavy textbook with all the plays and sonnets. A student hissed as I edged by, "Mummy, mummy, mummy," but I stared straight ahead. Mom scampered to the front and I followed, my face flaming. She tapped the seat beside her and looked at me with pleading eyes: "Stay with me!" I steeled myself for my last stand, and dumped her books on the desk. "No, Mom. I'd rather be at the back." Her face crumpled and I trilled with a guilt I would not acknowledge.

The professor, Dr. Black, bustled into the class and looked around. Did he wink at Mom? How disgusting! With the class list in his hand, he began to put faces to names. "Perry, Elizabeth." Mom hurled her hand into the air and shook it like a grade-one teacher's pet. "Perry, Janet." I twirled a tentative finger beside my ear, trying to look as if I didn't really care who I was. Dr. Black studied Mom, then studied me, then looked back and forth between us.

He cleared his throat. "Well, Miss Perry," he said, pointing to the desk I had refused to occupy moments before. "I want you right here." He waited while I moved. I sat. Mom smiled in triumph. He studied me. I looked down. "You need to help your mother," was all Dr. Black said.

I handled that badly, looking back at the experience from my maturity. What possessed me to make life so much harder for Mom than it already was? Why didn't I acknowledge the effort she was making to recover her life? But she couldn't acknowledge my feelings then, either. We never spoke about that part now, though we laughed about Dr. Black and No Fear Shakespeare and our time as students together. I would have given anything for a do-over of my behavior then. But perhaps that failure was part of the motivation to do better four decades later.

Now I had empathy for both Mom and Dad. I wished I didn't live three mountain ranges and a stretch of ocean away, a thousand miles and a time zone distant from the kind of help that was needed most. I worked to be present over the phone, but Dad couldn't hear and Mom said she didn't like to chat on the phone. Feeling isolated, I looked for ways to pitch in.

One way that was a real help to Judi was to deal with Goliath. It meant sitting on hold with Muzak and health messages, and being bumped from one office to another with one goal. Mom needed help at home. Judi hated being the daughter asking for it on behalf of her mother. There was always the implication, "Why don't you do it yourself?" My distance in this was power. Of course I could not vacuum or change the linen and scrub the tub, all things far beyond Mom's capability now. So while I waited on hold I read a book, kept up with my emails, but refused to be put off. Though it took months, Goliath agreed that Mom could have three hours a week of home care assistance.

I liked the name I gave the Alberta Health Services, in my head, of course. The Health Services I faced in my home province of British Columbia was just the same. I guessed that daughters all over North America, perhaps the Western World, might give the same nickname to their system. Did every bureaucracy have the same talent to tout the vision of the right to health care on the one hand while leaving the doubt that in reality it was being rationed somehow? I believed that Goliaths anywhere were blind giants, efficiently using guidelines, protocols and policies to keep users, we little Davids, in line. Judi said she appreciated me for taking the role of getting as much out of Goliath as possible, no matter how much effort it took.

Three hours of home care was not nearly enough for Mom. But it gave Judi three hours of freedom to do her own work. More important was the way having no glaring house care needs opened the way for Judi to spend that time as companion and daughter, not drudge. I was effusive in my thanks to the minion of Goliath that made the decision to support Mom this way.

Now on Monday, Wednesday and Friday, the home care aide arrived for exactly one hour. She rang the lobby buzzer, and at first Mom tried to lurch out of her recliner and limp with her walker to push the button near her door fast enough to let the person in before she left. They didn't wait long. Mom would tell me that they had not arrived and I would phone Goliath to report the absence and complain. Goliath would say that the client had not allowed access. What were they to do? Judi chewed nails when she heard this, and Mom whimpered that she just couldn't move fast enough. The only solution was to involve Judi, who waited every Monday, Wednesday and Friday for her buzzer to ring. Then she would leave her computer and whatever fleeting creative thought she might have been working through in that moment, and let the homemaker into the building. They seemed to change every week. When a new homemaker arrived, Judi hung around to show her the ropes, and talked to Mom for a few more minutes to observe how the homemaker was doing. There had been some problems that Mom called "situations." Once a home-maker with tired eyes and no English tried fruitlessly to plug the vacuum hose into the electrical outlet. Judi explained how plugs worked. On another occasion, Mom reported that lunch had been a spoonful of concentrated cream of mushroom soup, cold. "It looked like dogfood," she said. We laughed, but it was sad too. These women, new arrivals to Canada, were desperate for work, and Goliath was desperate for anyone who would accept work at the lowest end of the pay scale. When Judi found a homemaker in the bedroom on her cell phone, she was prepared to fire the unfortunate woman on the spot. "No," said Mom, "my guess is that she has her own mother to attend to while she is attending to yours." Incom-petence wasn't the biggest concern, though. Judi monitored for respect and honesty and an absence of abusive behavior towards Mom. Fortunately for Mom, there were only two or three times that she reported being handled roughly, or yelled at, or called stupid. Those women didn't get a second chance. We all agreed that some ineptitude was acceptable. But fear? No way! When Judi said a homemaker needed to be removed, getting that done was my job. I handled it with kid gloves. This was not just to avoid ruining the job prospects of needy people who might have had a bad day, but to avoid paperwork. Goliath was hyper-alert to abuse or threats of abuse, and any accusation resulted in a tangle of red tape. Small matters would lead to subtle shaming. Did I know how many frail elderly seniors without any family there were? Did Mom have any family close by who could help? Or why didn't she just hire a homemaker on her own?

The best help were the women who saw the main part of caregiving as caring. They tended to ignore Goliath's check-list of what to do for Mom around the house, and just ask her what help she really needed in the moment. In the long list of so-so assistants, there were a few of these. Like Cheryl. She was Blackfoot, newly arrived in Calgary from her family home on a reservation deep in the foothills, and she said she liked to work with elders. I noticed the tattoo on her shoulder and she explained that it was a medicine wheel. It represented the four directions, she said, and reminded her always of how humans have spiritual, physical, emotional and mental aspects to their beings. Mom and Cheryl got along in a way that went far beyond any relationship Goliath was paying for. "A girl deserves a bit of luxury," Cheryl would say each time she followed someone into the building to save Judi a trip downstairs, and walked into Mom's apartment without knocking. "What is your pleasure today?" Mom usually only wanted one thing. A bath, Cheryl-style. Mom trusted her. Cheryl helped Mom from her La-Z-Boy to the tub filled with hot water and bubbles. She helped Mom out of her dressing gown and gently lowered her up to her neck in luxury. Then Cheryl did what work she was expected to do while Mom had the bliss of a long soak. At the end of the day, Mom put her initials beside those official jobs and the bath remained their little secret. One day Cheryl didn't come. I sat on hold on the phone for hours, trying to speak to the boss and find out if something had happened to Mom's friend.

"Where is Cheryl?" I asked when I was finally in touch with the right person.

"Confidential," was the reply.

"Tell me, what is so secret? Is Cheryl OK? My mother wants to know."

"There were problems with her work," was all I could learn. Bubble baths were over.

Maria Gutierrez was a refugee from the jungles of Guatemala who spoke no English beyond phrases like, "Hurt here?" or "You cold?" or "You want juice?" and, "Let us pray."

Maria saw Mom's spiritual hunger and so didn't give a moment's thought to anything on the checklist of jobs. They spent their hour huddled together, Mom in her La-Z-Boy, Maria on her knees holding her rosary and Mom's hand. "Hail Mary, full of grace…" they crooned in unison in English and Spanish. Alas, Maria didn't stay long, either. "Pay no good," she told me mournfully when I tracked her down and talked to her, packing groceries at a Safeway store. "So sorry." It was just a fact. Most employers paid more than Goliath did.

Ninko Tshering was also a refugee. She had arrived from Tibet years before and spoke passable English. When she came to Mom, she wore her Tibetan garb that Mom remembered from her own travels in Nepal. The long silk sleeves and black robe with the hand-woven apron could not have been more inappropriate for the homemaking tasks, but they were perfect for Mom. While Ninko bustled around, they chatted about dharma and karma and the Pope. "I love your mother," Ninko told me. "She is an old soul." At Christmas, Ninko said she would like to make a big batch of *momos* for Mom, and enough extra for all her friends and family, too. Mom had smacked her lips once, remembering how much she had loved eating those spicy boiled dumplings on her travels to Ninko's homeland. Mom wrote a cheque for Ninko to buy the ingredients and we all looked forward to a special lunch. On her last work day before Christmas, Ninko arrived with her two sons. Over the next three hours, the kitchen filled with steam and spicy smells as the dozens of dumplings were prepared. Alas, Mom's stomach turned at the first nibble, and the mountain of dumplings remained untouched. "No problem," soothed Ninko, "my family likes them, too." Mom said she should take them to her family, so the sons packed the leftovers with an eagerness that made Mom delighted, too. They trooped off with their Christmas dinner courtesy of Mom, offering her warm hugs and prayers for her continued good karma. "We are family now," said Ninko. Mom glowed with pleasure about it all.

The second time Ninko asked for a loan, I began to be concerned about what "being family" entailed. Mom admitted that she had already written some cheques to help with this or that Tshering family emergency. I was sorry when I had to phone Goliath and say that this homemaker was no longer meeting Mom's needs.

Goliath had cutbacks. Mom's homecare help was the first to go. We were sorry, but a little relieved as well. Mom said she had liked fresh sheets on the bed but hated her loss of control as strangers swept around her feet and cleaned her bathroom. She said she wanted someone she knew. She wanted Judi to hire Joanne.

Neither Judi nor I liked Joanne, and Mom was quick to say the dislike was mutual. Joanne saw Judi and me as bossy. But Joanne had been Mom's employee in the years of the corner office and helped Mom navigate the worst of office politics then. They had become friends and Mom trusted Joanne to say what she thought. Mom said that Joanne had turned up her nose at what she saw of Goliath's homecare, and offered to be Mom's helper if she ever needed it. "Get Joanne," Mom said. "You do it," Judi said.

Mom agreed that a job description would be helpful and some sort of contract that would keep the relationship on an even keel. I smiled, guessing that Mom might have remembered some of her management challenges along with her friendship with Joanne. I developed a list of the things that needed doing, like changing the bed and doing the laundry and cleaning the tub. Mom said she didn't need vacuuming the whole house, but I said it would be good to at least clean up the trail of ash and drips that went from her chair to the bathroom to the bedroom to the kitchen, the only parts of the apartment Mom occupied now. Lunch would be nice, Mom thought, and getting the dishes done. I added the job of keeping track of the fridge, clearing out what had turned green with mold and making a shopping list of what was needed. If Joanne worked out, everyone would win. Mom said she wanted to pay Joanne well, as a friend and companion as much as a homemaker and helper. I wrote in a draft agreement that would give Joanne five dollars an hour over the rate of Goliath's workers. I sent it by email and Mom said she was sure it would all suit Joanne just fine. We were all wrong.

It was our birthday. Judi's family and mine had all chipped in to buy us a night in a fancy spa an hour out of Calgary. Jamie, my son, and Judi's husband, Tom, promised to keep an eye on Mom if we promised to spend this night away thinking about ourselves and not Mom or Dad. We were keeping our promise. I think we were imagining our futures after the Parent Project, swirling glasses of wine as we enjoyed the huge Jacuzzi in the room, possibly by candlelight. I am sure that my cellphone's ring broke the magic of the moment as I lunged to answer it, fearing the worst on the home front.

"How dare you!" It was Joanne, and she was furious. "What the hell do you think you are doing?" She railed at the idea of a contract she would have to sign, a checklist telling her what to do, and most of all the pittance of pay I offered. "That is not what Betty wanted!" Joanne huffed that she was a professional not a scullery maid, would never accept that slave wage and who did I think I was? I got out of the Jacuzzi and shivered as I negotiated a new rate that was several dollars an hour higher. Joanne was mollified. She would consider it. She wished us a good night and hung up. I too snapped the cell phone shut. The mood was broken, and now Judi and I bathed in cortisol, not lavender bubble bath. We talked until dawn about all the frustrations of the Parent Project, when it was time to leave the hotel and get back into it.

Mom assured us she was delighted with Joanne. She needed a pal more than a clean fridge. Joanne brightened her day, not just her bathtub. Judi began to hint that Joanne was not doing what she'd been contracted for. "The ashtray is full of butts with lipstick that doesn't belong to Mom, and the sink is full of coffee mugs now. The sheets haven't been changed in a month." I promised to have a word with Mom, and then Joanne, on my next visit. "It can't come soon enough," Judi huffed. "I've got two women to clean up after now."

Mom's eyes grew steely as I outlined my concerns about Joanne. I watched, now nervous but fascinated, as the ash on her cigarette grew impossibly long and then toppled on to her lap. She brushed it aside, adding it to the grey circle around her chair. Judi studied her coffee cup, leaving this tricky conversation to me. We both knew, though, that we were at some sort of crossroads. Mom wanted our support. But she wanted her control. We had slipped on that. We had forgotten our place. Finally Mom spoke. "I am paying for Joanne," she began. "And if I want her to lie in the sunbeams on my floor and make angels in my dust balls, that's my business." I tried to focus on the contract and the job description. I tried to say how Joanne was not doing the work she was being paid for. Mom would have none of it. We could just tear up that contract. She would decide what she would do with Joanne and we would have no more part of it. Our talk was over. She wanted to be alone. We said good-bye and slinked back to Judi's apartment to have a beer or two, debrief about what had just happened, and lick our wounds. Joanne stayed. Judi added Mom's laundry to hers and changed the bed when Mom asked for help with that. She loaded the dishwasher while she made the morning coffee as she always did when Joanne was not around. We knew that the twins were a frequent subject when Joanne and Mom were together. But the fact was, Mom was back in charge and we knew it made Mom feel better.

Joanne quit after a few more months saying she had got a real job, and things went back to the way they were before. But Judi and I had learned a good lesson.

We swore we would not get caught in the middle again. That's why we were not enthusiastic when my brother Chris told us about a new Goliath policy, called self-managed care. He had heard about it from an employee. "Wow!" he gushed, "it is just what Mom needs right now!" He'd learned that Mom needed to be qualified for this, but if she met the criteria there would be an annual whack of money for her to use as she saw fit to get the help she needed. The hitch was, she would not be able to turn to Goliath for anything else after that. She would have to find the helpers, monitor them, and pay all the bills including all the complicated payroll extras, employment insurance and tax receipts.

Mom said she was proud of Chris and excited that he'd found the solution to getting her real help. Why had I missed it? Chris said he would get Mom all signed up, but we would have to do the day-to-day administration on Mom's behalf. He was sure we'd do a fine job running self-managed care for Mom.

For the next several weeks, Chris mumbled about Goliath. What inscrutable rules it had! What complicated forms! What nosy requirements for personal financial information! He said he hated the taped music on hold and the health messages. I stayed silent, smiling to myself. Chris was getting a reality check about how difficult it was to work with the system. Perhaps, Judi and I agreed, he might be more sympathetic about what it took us to be the surrogates for Mom and Dad.

"God is good." Judi was as relieved as I was. Chris had phoned me, dejected. Mom had been rejected for self-managed care. It was for people who were really disabled, he reported, not merely living with multiple chronic problems and dwindling of old age, struggling to stay out of an institution. Mom didn't fit the policy. At least, we agreed, we would not be getting into personnel relations any more. Joanne had been enough.

A few months later, though, I fell for Goliath's dream again. I'd found a notice that a Family Caregivers Support Centre was opening with a mandate to back up the unsung heroes of the health care system, family caregivers. We could turn to the centre for resources and, even better, a sympathetic ear, a way to share what was poetically presented in the website as "the joys and sorrows of family caregiving."

Judi mocked me for my eagerness. Goliath had a new innovation every week, she said. Support zeroed in on family caregivers was new though, and she was intrigued to see what that might be all about. She was glad to come with me to check out this office just a few blocks from Hull Estates. I made an appointment for an information visit on my next trip to Calgary. I imagined how we would sign up for a workshop or two, a support group maybe, and perhaps befriend or be befriended by that Goliath employee that Judi just called "the sympathetic ear." The waiting room was empty when we arrived. It was furnished with plastic chairs and decorated with health-message posters and three rubber tree plants that needed water. Steel shelving was overstuffed with brochures from businesses offering something for sale. On the other side of a glass barrier, the woman I assumed was our contact studiously ignored us. A half hour went by. "Should we tell Dad we might be late?" I wondered. We were taking him to an eye specialist appointment after meeting with "sympathetic ear" and he had anticipated it for months. Dad must not miss this chance to have his glaucoma checked.

"Good idea," Judi agreed. "We sure don't want him standing in the wind on the corner to wait, he'll get frostbite." I punched in Dad's number and knew in an instant there was a problem. Dad shouted into the phone, "Who is it?" saying I must speak up, he couldn't hear. Dad wasn't wearing his expensive hearing aids. So I shouted. Judi put her fingers to her lips. The sympathetic ear's head snapped up and she stormed out to confront us. Couldn't we see she was busy? What was this racket? I steamed with embarrassment and anger. "We have an appointment," I sputtered, explaining about Dad and his hearing and how cold it was for an old man waiting outside in the wind, and how we were tight for time. Without apology, the woman pointed to a prominent sign with its list of reasons why people would be evicted from the Family Caregiver Support Centre. Then she said we would have to wait our turn, and went back to her office with a flourish. She had only one question for us. "Are you twins?" I was finished with sympathetic ear. We never went back.

It took many more months before I was ready to try another Goliath program. This one was too good to miss. Over four weeks, we family caregivers would learn some skills to help do our jobs more confidently. Participants were even offered a substitute caregiver as backup because, of course, family caregiving responsibilities would not stop while we learned about them. Judi and I almost danced to the first class. It was twin time, and we would learn something, too.

The first afternoon was about blood pressure. We learned everything there was to know about the numbers.

After coffee break we practiced on each other. "Any questions?" the instructor asked.

I raised my hand. "How would we interpret the results?" The instructor gave me a perplexed look and considered the question. "You write it in your caregiver's notebook and share it with the doctor on your loved one's next appointment."

The second afternoon we learned about how to give medications. We practiced how to crush pills and hide them in applesauce and keep them sorted and write down what should be taken when in the same journal we used for our blood pressure findings.

"Any questions?"

I raised my hand. "What do I do if my mother or father chokes on a pill?"

The instructor studied her watch. "That is a question for a whole other class," she said. "We don't have time in this session to get into that. I guess you would just thump him or her on the back."

The third afternoon we learned about waste management. We were told about constipation and diarrhea, haemorrhoids and impactions. On a suitably draped doll, we were told about inserting suppositories and giving enemas. After coffee break, we practiced putting diapers on a rubber doll that rolled over conveniently like I knew Mom never would.

"Any questions?"

I raised my hand. "How do we manage our gag reflexes?"

"You will get used to it." The instructor was soothing but clearly impatient with me. "It all sounds worse than it is."

The last day we learned how to heave our loved ones around without hurting them. 'Transferring', it was called. 'One-person assist'.

"Any questions?"

I raised my hand. "How can we protect our own backs?"

"I'll make a note of that," the instructor said. She agreed it should be part of the curriculum but admitted it wasn't yet. "Good question."

At the end of the course there were only three participants left from the dozen who had begun: Judi and me, and Mary. The rest had pleaded they were too busy caregiving to come to the classes. Mary had defeated-looking eyes and sighed when she spoke. She always wore a smock with a Winnie-the-Pooh motif and said she loved all its pockets. Her husband George had a stroke and was bedridden and crotchety. She said there was lots of help available for George, but it was the first time she found anything targeted to her needs. I suggested we celebrate our graduation as knowledgeable family caregivers at Starbucks. Mary demurred. That was impossible. George was waiting. So we hugged and promised to take a rain-check, but we knew that would never happen. As Mary left she turned around and said, "I wish I had a twin. I feel so alone."

"She's headed for burnout, sure as shootin'," Judi jabbed me as she waved good-bye.

8

Burn Out!

"We should..."

From my caregiver easy street on the Coast, I worried about Judi. Her temper was hair-trigger now, and when we talked on the phone, I seemed always to need to bring her down from what she downplayed afterwards as her tizzies. She couldn't get to sleep or stay asleep. She reached for what she called her brewskis as soon as she sat down to watch the news with her husband. It was light beer, she said, not much booze in it she assured me, and they calmed her down. She was sure of that. She admitted, though, that there were times when she had a lot of them. Then she warned me to lay off preaching to her. Of all people, I knew what she was up against. We code-named the situation of always having something to do for Mom or Dad the 'hamster wheel'. I could sometimes ask, "How is it spinning?" and sometimes she would laugh. But mostly, she said that harder she ran, the faster the darn wheel moved, and she had no clue how to get off it any more. We both knew that the wheel wouldn't stop for as far ahead as we could see. Both Mom and Dad were in a slow slide. Yet there was nothing that was, as the doctors put it, "a terminal diagnosis." Caregiving at this frantic whirl could go on for years. Judi compared it all to a game of whackamole in which she could bang one pop-up down if she was lucky, only to have another pop up somewhere else. Once Judi said aloud the thing she could hardly admit to herself. "I wish they would get on with it and just die." Shaken, I consulted Dr. Google. The wise old search engine confirmed my fears. Judi had a full blown, and dangerous, case of burnout.

One of the phrases Mom used that always amused both Judi and me was, "We should." It carried a world of meaning, but essentially was a way Mom had of pleading for help without admitting she needed it. Both of us had got used to jumping at "we should." She would say afterwards, "How did you know?" wondering if we could read her mind. We liked to think that this was her way of saying thank you, and "we should" was her substitute for please. Did other parents do this? Did other daughters fall right into the trap?

One job I could do from my distance was to record best seller books which were not available on audiotapes in the public library. For me, reading to Mom was a wonderful way to connect. But there was a problem. Dozens of used audiotapes piled up in Calgary after she had listened to them and needed to be returned for re-recording. Judi was having a particularly trying week when Mom said, "We should recycle those cassettes back to Janet."

Before she knew it, and certainly before she could contain it, Judi's volcano of pent-up anger erupted. "Do you really mean 'we', Mom?" Judi seethed. "When you say 'we' it's just another job for 'me', isn't it, Mom?" In tears when she phoned me that night, Judi said she would give anything to pull that moment of fury back. I tried to reassure her. Mom was far too mature to over-react to something so trivial as that one snap.

But was she? I knew that pressure was building in Mom, too. She hated feeling needy. And she knew that she needed more and more help from Judi. I knew Mom was having problems accepting her vulnerable situation. As Judi and I talked about this new trouble, I heard the telltale snap and fizz of a beer can being opened. How many was that? The thought flitted across my mind. I didn't dare ask.

With more snaps and fizzes the next night, Judi said how she had gone to Mom's apartment that morning with a peace offering of fresh coffee and the Scrabble board. She found Mom sitting in the dark, curtains drawn, the television black. Her voice was flat, Judi said, defeated.

"What's wrong, Mom?" Judi asked.

"Nothing. I am moving to assisted living in Timbuktu. I won't bother you anymore."

Mom's bipolar swings didn't worry me much anymore. Though she'd had them all her life, I'd finally figured them out as an adult and come to terms with them as a constant in Mom's personality. In her words, "It is what it is." But Judi was my concern. Would humour help? "Sure, moving Mom out of your sight forever would be just one more item in your job jar, Judi!" She didn't laugh.

She said she was getting another beer. I waited. Judi did not return to the phone. Where was she? In my mind's eye I saw the dangling receiver and my heart began to beat in a panic I couldn't pinpoint. My imagination took me to her 25th-floor balcony, though. I hated that balcony myself, hated looking over the edge to the street so far below. Could Judi have just heaved herself over the edge, I wondered? All night I dialed and redialed Judi's number, getting nothing but a busy signal. She just wasn't there. Finally, in my pre-dawn frenzy on the West Coast, Judi answered, surly, with a slight slur. "What's up?"

"You are alive!" I sputtered. "You didn't jump!"

"What in God's name are you talking about?" She said I was being ridiculous. Who did I think she was? Yes, she had gone to the balcony. It was a lovely sunset. Yes, she must have forgotten the phone off the hook and me waiting for her at the other end. "Sorry," she said, sounding impatient. But she said her concern was not leaving me hanging, but Mom. She had forgotten I was on the line, but she'd fallen asleep and missed her last visit to say good night to Mom. It was her regular drop-in at Mom's bedtime that we all called the 'tuck-in'. Had Mom worried when Judi didn't appear for the tuck-in, or was she just relieved that Judi had understood how she needed time alone?

I obsessed all day about Judi and Mom and things falling apart with Martha and Dad, too. At Dad's seniors' residence, the "in sickness and in health" part of Martha's marriage vow to Dad seemed to have less pull now. She said she was worn down. "Family has to take care of him, I can't." Was Dad a package to be returned to sender somehow when he didn't meet expectations? She sighed once, talking to me, "I didn't get the best years of your father." It wasn't complaining, just the way it was with her. Actually, Martha was a test of my compassion, and I failed it with flying colours, seeing red!

The next morning, after a sleep-disturbed night with dreams of balconies, I began to write. Through all the times of tumult in my life, I'd kept a journal. Writing and ripping was my way to corral the chaos of my thoughts. Usually seeing my emotions converted to ink took the edge off them, too. I reached for a pen now, turned off the computer and the phone, and scribbled all morning. For a while I rambled through diffuse anxiety and anger about how all-encompassing this parent care had become. I examined what the phrases, 'multiple complex conditions' and 'dwindling in old age' actually added up to in terms of Judi's front-line obligations, and mine more distant, though only in terms of miles. Eventually I decided to harness my angst in a letter. "Dear Judi," I began.

"Now I'm scared! I can't bear to think of you falling apart. My mind assures me you are strong and would never take a dive from the twenty-fifth floor. But last night my nightmares said otherwise. Just those thoughts leave me helpless and feeling terrified. When we talked yesterday you kept saying, 'It's OK', and just as screwball, 'It's nothing'. That's not true, Judi! This hamster wheel is spinning out of control. Just add up all you do and it's obvious. I organized my thoughts around 'doctoring A to Z'. Would it help at least to name the problem?

"**Audiologist** – Dad is always fiddling with his digital hearing aids, cranking them up, winding them down. They cost a frigging fortune and yet they aren't worth a damn. They whistle all the time. Why can't the audiologist figure it out? Why does she tell you what Dad needs to do, when he's sitting right there in front of her? The truth is, I guess, that Dad's brain is too old to deal with the kind of hearing loss he has. His frustration with those gizmos, and the audiologist with him, spills all over you.

"**Cardiologists** – Between Dad and Mom's tricky tickers, you've got a lot of appointments to set up, drive to, sit with, follow-up on. Dad's heart races even when he's sitting in his chair. Is his pacemaker broken? Mom's heart beats too slowly. I hate it when she starts feeling her pulse, her brow furrowed.

'What's wrong?' I ask and she whimpers, 'Nothing, dear'. Is that what makes her feel so dead to the world all the time?

"**Dentists and Denturists** – One blessing is that Mom's teeth are still holding up, even though she doesn't brush often or floss ever. But Dad's dentures? His choppers are a disaster. I've found them in his bedclothes, under the bed, in the toilet once. He tells me he can't get them to stick. Do you notice his drools of Polident?

"**Dermatologists** – Why does Dad scratch? And what's with those red blotches up and down Mom's arm? She's sure it's more skin cancer. She's had so many lesions taken off already. The doctor says it's just a bruise and old people get them and to stop fussing. But Mom says her skin crawls and feels like it is on fire and it's just weird. Dr. Nan just shakes her head and says, 'Weird skin is not a symptom, Betty'. Is it post-shingles pain?

"**Endocrinologists** – Dad's lady breasts are because of his low testosterone. Martha says she's happy that he's running out of juice because it makes him less frisky, finally! You said his family doc just chuckles about that. He says Dad's got a lot of miles on him and has to expect to wear out. Do you think underneath that doctor's smile is his ageism? You know, 'horny old goat'.

"But Mom? What she calls, in her nurse lingo, 'brittle diabetes' might spell the end for her living at home. Testing her blood is the easy part, but even that just makes her crazy. Sugars are over the top one hour on that infernal meter that always asks her for more blood while she stabs away at herself, and then an hour later they have tanked. I hear you. Insulin shots would mean the end of living at home. I wonder…would that be so bad?

"**Gastroenterologist** – I hate that kidney bowl always on Mom's lap. Her nausea is awful for both of you since you are the clean-up girl. Don't let me get going on the poop problems! Can't shit. Can't stop shitting. Speaking of clean-up, that's the really disgusting chore. You downplay it, too, though, thinking more of Mom's dignity to have to admit to an accident and watch you on your knees. I wonder if it is time for diapers?

"**Gerontologists, or not** – Why does every doctor think there is nothing special about looking after the ills of the elderly? My guess is, they hate to see Mom or Dad coming into their office. Neither of them gets in or out of an appointment in the ten minutes they get paid for by Goliath. Bet the docs are happy to see you, though. Helping with the dressing and undressing, asking the questions, taking the notes, overseeing the follow-up. All that is probably the most important thing you do for their well-being as far as doctoring goes.

"**Oncologists** – What a twisted world! Dad being relieved to hear he has blood cancer because at least it explains why he feels so awful. But then the battle with Shady Pines. You said it is a union thing. Staff refuse to handle a body leaking radioactive tinkle after a chemo treatment. How can they refuse to care for Dad? Does it mean all folks with cancer can't be treated and still stay in assisted living? I guess it's lucky that it didn't become a showdown after all, thanks to dad refusing any more chemo. But blood transfusions are no better. They knock the poor guy out. Dad told me the doctor called it a lazy cancer? Means I guess that he'll be alive with it, but sentenced to the wheelchair because he's so totally out of gas. And Mom's so-called chronic lung cancer? Of course it's good news that her lung nodules don't seem to grow or shrink or spread. 'You will die with this cancer, but not of this cancer'. Remember how the doctor said that last time we were with her at an appointment? But she's not really free of it, is she? I'm sure that oxygen tank she's attached to now is going to do her in sooner or later. She'll trip on the tube and break her hip, or more likely blow herself to smithereens lighting a cigarette too close to the tank.

"**Nephrologist** – Do Mom's kidneys still ooze pus in her piss? 'No big deal', the doctor said. 'Almost all old ladies have urinary tract infections'. But a common problem doesn't make it a small one, does it? She has to endure the stinging and aching and dribbling and stinking for the rest of her life. Poor Mom. Poor you.

"**Neurologists** – How many mini-strokes have sent you to Emergency with Dad?

"**Orthopedists** – With everything else going south, it's Dad's big toe he complains about the most! It must really hurt. Why can't anyone just fix that one little thing? 'Just arthritis?' That's no answer! But nothing bone-wise Dad can complain about can beat how fast Mom's spinal stenosis is crumbling her body. Did you know that Dr. Google says that might develop into paralysis?

"**Ophthalmologists** – Macular degeneration changed everything for Mom. Frankly, I am glad she isn't getting those shots in the eyeball anymore. That doctor was really honest, telling her he couldn't in good conscience take her money anymore because the drug wasn't making a difference. So she's destined to have that big black blot in both eyes now. On the bright side, if there can be one, Dad's glaucoma has not led to blindness so far. By the way. We do that, don't we Judi...hasten to 'look on the bright side?' I think optimism is one of our gifts, don't you? His aim with those expensive drops is lousy, though. Each drop dribbling down his cheek is another few bucks. Martha says she's tried to help but he tells her to scram, he'll manage himself. Drip, drip, drip. It's the fine line, isn't it, this balancing act between staying independent and being incompetent. But if one of the cute nurses at Shady Pines could take it on? Dad might like one of them scrunching his face!

"**Psychiatrists** – Dad's sunny ways persist through every new challenge. Is it his belief that God is in charge, or his gift of optimism? A mix, I think. I've seen him morose on visits, but he bounces back. He's dodged the bullet of the really bad blues so far. But Mom? She maintains depression is normal in the elderly. I'm guessing her bipolar condition is getting worse. More downs than ups now, though.

"**Pain Specialist** – Dr. Spanswick is a hero. Remember how we had to advocate to get her in to see him the first time? Goliath kept saying her pain problem was low priority, because she was not in the work force. She'd just have to wait in the non-urgent lineup. When I finally got to him through all his gatekeepers, he acted right away. 'Nonsense!' he said. 'It's the folks with a short time left on this planet that are my top priority.' I could have kissed him. And from that first treatment, Mom was much better. It was sad when he said he couldn't safely inject more cortisone into Mom's spine. So now it's only the opiates. Do you think Mom is hooked on morphine? They say no, not if she's not faking the pain. But I'm sure those drugs are what are making her so foggy so much of the time. She can't win!

"**Urologist** – Dad can't pee, Mom can't stop peeing. Say no more! I think Dad has some Viagra in his wallet still."

When I was done with randomly listing all of the medical woes, it was starkly obvious why Judi was wearing out. She was the force behind every doctor visit from the setting up of the appointments to the driving and listening and following up with the inevitable labs and X-rays and sending in a sample of this or that. There was all the rest of it, too. Drug management. Judi had to be on top of everything, making sure no pill ran out. Picking up the prescriptions, watching for side effects, figuring out when Dad or Mom must take each pill and what other pill must not be taken at the same time and whether it was milk to be avoided or grapefruit juice. What pill could be crushed? What must be taken whole? She was a pharmacist without the title.

And all the non-doctoring jobs. Helping keep bills paid, keeping an eye on their minuscule investments, each with its separate report, gathering the receipts to get whatever tax deductions might be lurking in the fine print. Being financial manager was an unsung aspect of keeping an eye on things.

I found myself getting tired just adding up the hours, thinking of Judi also struggling to maintain her life, as oldsters she loved sucked her dry without her even being aware of it. Neither would stop getting old. There was no end in sight.

I signed off, trying to decide whether it was "in admiration" or "in sympathy" or "sadly" or "with regret." How did I feel about all this? So I didn't send the letter. Instead, I phoned Judi and she sat patiently on the other end of the line, with more snap and fizz, while I read the litany. Then we talked, about her this time. What could she do for herself, to save her sanity?

Judi took it seriously. After our call, she found a counsellor who understood the pressures she was under but also pushed her. She must attack the problem that was not about her parents but herself. She must reframe her situation as a caregiver enough to reclaim her life beyond that. The counsellor agreed that caregiving might go on for years, but forced Judi to accept how it would not be forever. So Judi needed strategies to train her mind to think in a different way. What was the best she could do in the moment? That must be good enough, the counsellor insisted. I was relieved when Judi took that on. But as always with Judi, she took on her new commitment to herself in a grand scheme. "I'm going to do a marathon." In six months, she said, she would join a group raising money for leukemia and lymphoma research and walk 26 miles around the streets of Phoenix. To train for it, she would be out every day with the other marathoners and a coach. Would I help her raise funds for this? She wanted to raise at least a few hundred dollars as she raised her spirits and fitness level. I was delighted. Here was something we could both dive into, me on the Coast and her in Calgary and, best of all, it was about something other than parent care. When Judi was finished walking that January day, she was proud of her accomplishment and we both knew she would not let her body slip back into its old ways.

After the near miss of burnout, I turned a corner, too. Now I made a point to visit Judi in Calgary when she was not headed out on business travel leaving me in charge. We took a vacation together, to an all-inclusive resort while my husband stayed behind to do the parent care. We slept till noon, sat by the pool in the afternoon, strolled along the beach to watch the sunset, and watched old movies in our room till late into the night. We kept our promise to check our emails no more than once a day, talk about other things than Mom and Dad.

We returned refreshed, and the next year did it again. Just as Judi's counsellor had foreseen, this Parent Project could go on for years.

Back on the Coast, I became a different kind of retiree than I had been before. I gave up on any thoughts of starting a second career and did not pursue contract possibilities. Instead, I filled my agenda with volunteer activities. They had been satisfying in many ways, but they had also become obligations to serve, and drags on my time and tranquility. Now, aware of my own risk of burnout, I changed my pattern and backed out of as many commitments as I could. I avoided all the temptations to take new leadership roles and became an "I will if I am free" kind of volunteer. I took up yoga, and began to meditate and walk solo or with friends along the many trails. I joined a book club of supportive women and we all became intimate friends with each other as we got to know the fiction section of the library. I realized over the next months that what Judi and I still called "the balcony scene," had been a turning point. Both of us were better equipped now to face the potential of a long haul as caregivers. Life in Calgary stayed busy. But it was more peaceful now.

9

Crash!

"I live in hope."

I relaxed. The sound of sloshing water told me Mom managed to get into her bath without help. She needed a long soak. The family reunion around Dad's birthday, and Steve's annual storm blowing into Calgary from Africa with his children and to-do list, was over. It was wonderful, but it took every ounce of energy we had. Whew! Judi and I were the main organizers. Did we take that role or were we given it? I didn't know. We called it duck work. Our twin feet paddled furiously under the surface while the observer would only see serenity. We liked that lie. Once Judi was back from dropping the last load of visitors at the airport, we would get into the wine and the beer and debrief on Mom's balcony. Mom might join our very happy hour, but I hoped she would choose bed. I wanted twin time.

Wow! Dad was 90! He looked his age. He was out of gas for anything more than cupcakes and tea in the common room with anyone who wanted to drop by. As usual, Martha said it was up to family to organize a celebration. That was OK. We didn't want her meddling. Dad's speech was the highlight, everyone said. Martha said he'd been in a tizzy about it for weeks, saying it over and over, unable to remember a single word. My sister Nancy soothed his jitters and led him lovingly to the microphone saying, "You can do it, Dad. Just be yourself." So he was. He rambled about his boyhood, oozing spittle when he laughed at his own memories, losing his place on his wad of script, and starting over again. I noticed that all the other oldsters had fallen asleep, heads sagged on chests or lolled to the side, and there was the hum of snoring. I signaled to Nancy to wind it up. Dad protested that he had ten pages more to go, but with the special touch that only Nancy really had with Dad, she prevailed. As we scraped the gobs of icing off the floor, we marveled at how dementia had not defeated our father. He was actually more endearing as he lost that short-fuse edge and the emotional distance he'd cultivated all our lives. I was grateful that he still remembered all our names. There were no guarantees how long that would last. Would he still know us by the next family reunion?

Steve turned 45 the next day and had told Judi and me to prepare a picnic at Sandy Beach. It was a happy place in all our childhoods. Steve thought our efforts to keep Dad away from Mom were ridiculous. If they had a feud it was theirs to manage. Judi and I agreed it was all childish on one level, but we also knew there was something deeply disturbed in Mom to have her so adamant that she could not, would not, reconcile. Her feelings were her business. But looking at Dad now, slumped in a wheelchair, I wondered how he could still manipulate. What I knew for sure was that I didn't want a blow-up at the party.

It was a picnic to remember. There was an intergenerational baseball game. Hide and seek. More food than any of us could consume and beer, too, in paper cups because this was a public park. Mom relaxed when Dad left, tired and pale, and then became that part of manic we all loved. When Mom was happy, we all were. The memories of the weekend mixed in my mind with happy memories of childhood.

Crash! A strangled cry. I ran to the bathroom. Mom sprawled on her back, naked and moaning. Her breasts flopped to both sides of her now-prominent ribs. Her gnarled hands, covered in deep red bruises, tried to cover herself, so my first move was to put a towel over her body. "Oh Mom!" I fell to my knees beside her, reaching under her armpits to help her up.

"My back is broken!" she howled, and I leaned back on my knees to consider while she cried, "I know it is broken, I can feel it." I speed-dialed Judi, driving along the Deerfoot freeway from the airport. "Call 911." Her voice was clipped, tense. This was all my fault. How could I have left Mom to get out of the tub on her own? But how could she have tried that without asking for help?

The sound of the ambulance screaming to a halt at the front door of the apartment brought out all the neighbours, who hung over their balconies to see. I waved and hollered, "Up here," and ran to the elevator to usher the ambulance crew to Mom's side. The young paramedic felt her body up and down. "No obvious broken bones, Ma'am," he assured her. He turned to me. "She needs an X-ray, though. We'll take her to Emergency."

"What's the lineup like?" I asked.

The paramedic sighed. "It's a summer long weekend, Ma'am, what can I say?" I knew Mom had to go, however long the wait. I packed the Emergency Room bag with the supplies I knew we would need: the eye mask, the ear plugs, the bottle of water with a straw, the sour candies for the dry-mouth time. Where were the mouth swabs? Where was her shawl? What about her talking book and extra batteries? Her rosary? I knew what we needed after long experience.

Every plastic chair was occupied by groaning or stoic people when the paramedic pushed Mom's stretcher into the waiting area reserved for higher-status ambulance arrivals. People stood around and leaned against the walls and stood outside the doors to smoke, but I noticed the daughters, holding the hands of their suffering parents, clearly uncomfortable on their ranks of unforgiving chairs. The triage nurse was stone-faced. She pointed to a corner and told me, "Sit her over there." I reached for my advocate's hat, a helmet really. It was tough to face down this gatekeeper.

"No, she stays on her stretcher," I glared. "She has injured her back. She can't sit. So she must lie flat until the doctor sees her." The nurse held my eyes for a moment or two until I saw her expression soften. Did she see her own mother in mine? Was this the daughterhood effect operating? Did Goliath have a guideline to avoid incidents with bitchy daughters losing it and creating a rumble that might get into the news as elder abuse?

"Just this once," she said.

"Thank you," I replied with a smile I hoped looked as grateful as I really was.

Judi and I took turns holding Mom's hand. When it was Judi's turn, they said the rosary. When it was mine, I read the editorial page of the Calgary Herald, and the world news. When Mom said she just craved sleep, we put the blackout mask over her eyes and fit the spongy plugs in her ears. Then we relaxed to doze ourselves. We knew the routine.

In the wee hours of the next day, a young man with a white coat bustled in, studying a clipboard. Without much conversation beyond, "How did this happen?" he felt Mom head to foot. "Hurt here? Hurt here? Hurt here?" Then he shined a penlight into her eyes and asked her to follow the light. "No concussion. Nothing broken," he confirmed. "She's going to be very sore for a few days, there are big bruises." He gave me a packet of Extra Strength Tylenol, and Judi laughed.

"Is that all you've got, Doctor? She eats these for breakfast." He looked at her strangely. I imagined he had put us all into the drug-seeking category.

"See your family doctor." He patted Mom's hand peremptorily, hurled the curtain aside, and was gone. The nurse pointed to the wall phone and said we could get a taxi. Mom was discharged. Back went my advocate helmet. "No. Please arrange for non-urgent patient transfer. We will wait." I knew in refusing to leave we were bed-blocking now, but our twin team was something fierce. There was no way we could let Mom be dumped from the system without a way to get home lying flat. We would not budge until we got what Mom needed. I thought of the crowded waiting room and the other suffering mothers outside. I didn't dwell on that. Mom's comfort was my job. Bed-blocking was our best strategy.

"For God's sake! Get her an ambulance then!" Under her breath the nurse added, "Just get them the hell out of here." As we wheeled away, she whispered, "Your mother is lucky to have you." I smiled. It was the daughterhood.

The paramedics plopped Mom on her bed at an awkward diagonal and left her saying, "Give her some Tylenol before you try to straighten her out." They had no time to wait for that. There was no painkiller potent enough to keep

Mom from shrieking as Judi and I, kneeling on either side of her on the soft queen mattress, tried desperately to budge her dead weight with a "One, two, three, heave!" So we left her sprawled where she was, and stuffed bath towels between her legs. "Let it rip, Mom," I said. "You can't get to the toilet, it's OK to soak them. We'll do a wash." Over the next two days as she lay immobile and groaning, we fed her meal replacements through a straw. We stayed upbeat, but called Mom's friend and family doctor, Nan, to please come by as soon as she could. Dr. Nan's face showed no emotion as she wrote a prescription for a stronger version of morphine than Mom had ever had. When she slept, we huddled in the kitchen over coffee and talked about what was next. Dr. Nan said this immobility would bring more problems the longer it went on. Mom needed Community Nursing care. She made a call and left a message. "I'll arrange it." Then she told us that this would be a tough patch for Betty, and that a hospital bed would make it easier. That and a commode and a pole for Mom to grip, because we must force her to get up. The biggest challenge would be to keep her bowels open and her skin from breaking down. It's simple nursing care, she added, but you have to do it right. "Bring her in to see me in a month."

We called the paramedics again. Would they help us move Mom from her queen-size bed to the hospital bed we had rented and set up in the living room. "Is she on the floor?" the dispatcher asked.

"No," I replied, and explained the problem of moving her.

"Sorry, Ma'am," the operator said, "our people can pick up seniors who have fallen on the floor, but we are not authorized to move them from one place to another."

"You mean we have to push her out of the old bed to help her into the new one?" I was astounded.

"Our people are not authorized—" I hung up.

Fortunately, a neighbour was willing to help with the "hip-hike shift," and though Mom screamed it was done quickly. Now we were all more comfortable. I phoned my husband.

"I'm stuck here for a while," I said. "No, I have no idea when I will be home." I could hear the resignation in his voice, with a hint of impatience and even overtones of bitterness.

"Hurry back," was all he said. "I need you, too."

"I'll call you every day," I replied. Part of the success of the Parent Project was our husbands. They knew to just let us be.

We became "my little nurses." That's what Mom called us. She even called for us, "Nurse! Nurse!" when she needed something. I assumed it was the fog of morphine. Ten days passed in this blur of pain and boredom and fear.

Mom had gone many days without "moving her bowels," as she put it in better days. She could not manage the commode. Jugs of prune juice had no effect other than to give her cramps. The nurse said it was the morphine and immobility. Mom was getting an impaction, she suspected, but there were a few more things to try. She handed me a package of suppositories and an enema. "Use this."

Judi recoiled. "No way!" She was a daughter, not a little nurse, and she'd had enough of this whole thing. The community nurse was firm. "Then you will have to hire a private nurse. And you will be surprised how much that costs. Better to get over being prissy. Here, let me show you this time."

"I'll do it," I said. "It's no big deal." The nurse patted Mom's hand as she winced. It was a big deal. Mom was a supremely private person and this was the biggest affront to her dignity that she had yet endured. She squeezed her eyes shut as if that would make it all go away.

"You need to get your mother on to the list for long-term care," the nurse said as she packed her gear to leave, still without any toilet success for Mom. Goliath faced a long line of frail elders just like Mom, all waiting to be assessed. It was important to get into that line, because Mom would not be getting better now. Sure, the bruises would heal. But her back had been jerked in a way that would mean more pain in future. It was falls that spelled the end most often for the very elderly. "She's very frail."

I did my best with the bowel care, and I got used to the procedure as the nurse had assured I would. Nothing budged. It was the 13th day and Mom clutched her stomach with cramps and vomited. The impaction was now an emergency. The visiting nurse called 911, and said, "I need to talk to you girls." She told us that she admired our pluck. Few people would go so long in the ambiguity that we faced with this. But we needed to be considerably less competent now if we were to get what Mom needed: her admission into hospital. "Cry as you arrive. Be hysterical. If Goliath sees you as capable daughters, your Mom doesn't stand a chance." She wondered if we would be able to just have the ambulance take her, and stay out of sight till Mom had been admitted. Elderly people without family got looked after faster. It was a heartless triage. We would have none of it. We talked while we waited for the door buzzer to ring saying the paramedics were back. There were no sirens this time. The nurse said that staff in emergency rooms described the elderly chronic visitors like Mom as frequent fliers. There was even a word, GOMER, which staff used as code. "Here comes another GOMER." It meant, "Get out of my Emergency Room," and who could blame Goliath's foot soldiers? With their plates already full of life-threatening problems, a GOMER was just a bother. We packed the emergency kit again.

The nurse was right. "Old lady can't poop" did not beat out the life and death needs in the emergency room that night. And there were daughters on hand. So it was not until sometime the following afternoon that Mom was admitted to a bed at the end of a long hall, given a powerful laxative and sleeping pill and told to wait. Exhausted but relieved that Mom was in safe hands, we left for a few hours' rest and a shower.

So Mom was alone when her dammed-up bowel burst. Turkey soup, she called the stinky goo that dripped off her bed like lava and pooled on the floor. She lay in it for an hour before her call bell was answered. "Good for you, Mrs. Perry!" the nurse said as she called the orderly to clean the mess.

We played the good news/bad news game often in our Parent Project. It softened tough situations and kept us grateful and optimistic. Mom had been in hospital for a week, and the bad news was she had a diagnosis of "advanced level of de-conditioning." But the good news was she was crapping nicely again. The bad news was that she was ready for discharge, long before any of us were ready to help her take on life at home again. The good news was that in these nightmare three weeks, Mom had beaten her lifelong smoking addiction. Every four hours, Judi and I had slapped on a new nicotine patch. Her body was covered with blotches, and gummy. But Mom was not saying any more, "Where are my cigarettes?" She said she was done with smoking. She admitted she missed the mouth feel of the cigarette, the warmth of the smoke going in and the rush when she exhaled. Her fingers needed something else to do. But she had new confidence in her ability to still make big changes in her life. Perhaps this was a sign of better things to come. "I live in hope," she claimed.

10

Optimism

"I just want to stay in my home."

Mom was in big trouble. "Old lady can't poop" had performed, and was being discharged from the hospital. She said she never felt more like just packing it in. How could she manage at home? On the other hand, how could she stay? Dr. Maria, the hospitalist, was sympathetic but firm. "Your mother is struggling, I know that," she said, "but she doesn't have the kind of problem that any hospital can fix. We are about curing the sick around here, not lodging them." Dr. Maria felt it was time for long-term care. Like it or not, it was the only place where she would get the simple but substantial nursing care she needed now. "I'll complete the forms you need." But nothing happened fast in Goliath's world. She'd have to manage at home for a while. Mom closed her eyes. In the long silence I wondered if she was asleep. Then, in a whisper she said, "I just want to stay in my home."

I almost missed the tiny article buried deep in Goliath's website. It was in a section headed something like "Future Thinking," and described a pilot program for fragile seniors leaving hospital. It was called The Geriatric Assessment and Rehabilitation Program or GARP. Its hyped magic was happening just two floors below where Mom lay now, apparently bed-blocking. The article proclaimed that inter-disciplinary care for the frail elder was the secret for success. GARP could pull seniors back from their brinks to spend more months or years living independently. Even better, GARP would save a bundle for Goliath, keeping these dwindlers out of emergency rooms and acute care settings in hospitals. Everyone would win with the GARP advantage, the article proclaimed. Judi shared my giddy delight, and so did Dr. Maria.

"Why have I never heard of this place?" Dr. Maria wondered. "Two floors away, for heaven's sake, and it might as well be on the other side of the moon! I send poor old folks like your mother packing every day without being able to offer anything, and yet there it is, just below me!" She referred Mom, and by the end of the day it was settled. Instead of going back to her La-Z-Boy until the next emergency, we wheeled her downstairs to a place we all called 'hope'. The Director and Principal Researcher greeted her. "Welcome to rehab boot camp," she said. "This place is no picnic, but when we are done, you will be a new woman." I hoped Mom would not have one of her bipolar mood plunges, a hissy fit over some requirement or other she didn't like, or refuse to stick with GARP's plan. I hoped Mom would find her courage and endurance, and embrace the program of GARP. Judi and I had no idea how this would work out. What we did know for sure was that we were desperate to see Mom get some life back. "Please God let GARP deliver—" I stopped myself. Praying? "Be well, Mom, be well," I muttered. That felt better.

Red lines every few meters measured out the distance of GARP's long hall. Large print affirmations lined the walls. It had the spirit of a gym, not a hospital ward. There was team spirit, too, a belief that these discouraged oldsters had good living ahead of them. I felt an instant affinity with the place. GARP was my salvation, not just Mom's second chance.

The director told Judi and me to stay away for a few days. Mom needed to settle in without anyone speaking for her. She would be seen by a string of specialists, and needed to get into the routines of her well-being. Eating three meals, sleeping when she was supposed to, and getting her crippled body moving were on her agenda. We celebrated our freedom by going to a movie that first night, a healing dose of twin time. When we were allowed back to visit, Mom was in a jolly mood. She regaled us with stories of all the people who had come by to see her. The pharmacist had concluded right away that all the pills had to go. Once she was 'clean', she said, they could rejig the medications to the ones she really needed. "Less is better around here," Mom said, "except for exercise. That part is over the top." She explained how a twenty-something girl with a nose ring had run her through a routine of moves she needed for the Activities of Daily Living. These were the two dozen exercises to tighten and build the muscles she needed to get in and out of bed, on and off the toilet, clothes on and off and so forth. She needed to do all those things to stay at home. The psychiatrist scoffed at her idea that depression was just one of the things about being old she had to accept. She needed goals! She needed a perspective overhaul! She needed hope! But the best part was Dr. Spanswick. He was the pain specialist who some months before had actually listened to her, actually done something that actually helped. When he bounced into her room saying she'd hit the jackpot with GARP, Mom said she felt like she'd died and gone to heaven. Mom's face did look radiant as she explained it all.

By the fourth day, things had changed. Mom grumbled that she was not having a good experience anymore. The nurse's aide had tickled her toes at an ungodly hour and forced her to eat oatmeal. The physiotherapist had forced her to walk the whole length of the hall. "I vomited, you know," Mom said. "I tried to tell them that I was going to vomit and they said they'd clean it up, just keep moving. Can you imagine?!" She did a lot of vomiting over the next few days. Finally she turned the corner and said the nausea was gone. And better than that, Mom even admitted the calisthenics were fun. She liked being with the other old biddies lifting broomsticks into the air and touching their toes to get their shoe-tying moves down pat. All this was done to the wartime beats of Vera Lynn. Mom was beginning to glow again.

Judi and I turned our attention to Dad. As Mom was getting a second wind in GARP, Dad was losing his spunk. He tried to be cheerful, of course, which was his way. But now, he couldn't sustain a smile for long. We visited every day. He said he hadn't seen us for months but thank God we were back. "My twins," he crooned. "Are you Judi or Janet?" We pushed him in a wheelchair for walks along the river and stopped for ice cream. We took him to Tim Hortons for a donut or two and a coffee. We helped him find his favorite Louis L'Amour cowboy books in the library. Dad said he read all day, but his bookmark never moved. Martha said he was going to have to move to an assisted-living facility. She couldn't handle him anymore at home.

Judi and I were working hard on the home front. A two-bedroom apartment had come available at Hull Estates, and Judi snapped it up. When Mom got home, she would need a live-in caregiver, and that person would need space. We grabbed the chance to go through her place looking for anything that was surplus in her diminished life. We shredded years of files. We sent a huge pile of her spiffy wardrobe from another time to the thrift store. One day I dumped Mom's silver box full of tangled necklaces from the Corner Office glory days, and separated all the bits of gold. "Sell it," Mom ordered, and I took it to Goldfinger and earned several hundred dollars. "Give it away," Mom ordered, and I did. We tried to put Mom's pictures and furniture in the new place the same way it was in the old. On every bit of art or kitsch, Judi and I stuck a label with a name. Someday Mom would have to give this all away. Judi wanted her to decide who would get what. I gave her the inventory. She didn't even look at it. "There's no U-Haul behind the hearse, you know," was all she said.

One happy GARP afternoon, the three of us described our dream live-in caregiver. She would need one. Well, Mom said, it would be a mature lady of any culture or religion, as long as she was knowledgeable about it and proud, but not pushy or yakky. Her perfect companion would back off instantly if Mom wanted to be alone, and just know that without being told. She would be right there listening, though, the instant Mom wanted to be social. She might whip up a poached egg here and there, brew some coffee or do a laundry. For Judi and me, this paragon's main job, though, was to be the first responder. We wrote all of this in a cheerful advertisement for Craigslist and bulletin boards everywhere. No money would change hands, but this was the best barter deal in town. The lucky lady would have a furnished bedroom in an upscale building, and use of a kitchen. There were two replies, "What does the job pay?" was the only question. The second bedroom stayed empty. "God will provide," Mom said. Was I being cynical? I whispered to Judi, "God sure will provide. He'll provide you and me."

That was the problem. I didn't want to live out of a suitcase in Calgary. I was restless, and frustrated by the day-in-day-out requirements as caregiver on deck. I wanted more than anything else to get back to my life on the Coast. I could stay just a little longer till Mom was out of GARP and settled in her recliner and back in business looking after herself. A month? I could do one more month. So I decorated Mom's second bedroom to my taste, and accepted the routine of the live-in caregiver.

I got to work to get the physical supports Mom would need after I was gone. I lined up Meals on Wheels. I endured the form-filling and sitting on hold on the phone, begging Goliath to offer more help to Mom. It was a miracle. She was given six hours a week of personal support. Judi and I rejoiced. This living independently dream might actually work! I ordered a pendant with a call button Mom could use in an emergency to get help. Mom said that was creepy. I said it was essential.

When Mom left GARP after six weeks, we cavorted to the car, Judi twirling Mom in her wheelchair and Mom saying how good the fall breeze felt, and how she could smell the leaves. I doubted that, but told her smelling anything was her prize for getting off cigarettes. We sang "You are my sunshine..." all the way home and weren't embarrassed. It was one of the happiest moments I'd had in the caregiving journey. The future looked bright.

Two opportunities popped up, both the same day. The first was a contract for Judi. It was a six-month gig to develop a communications strategy but required her to work from the company's office. Judi said she would have a free hand to be as creative as she liked. And the money was good. It was more than money, though, I knew. Judi needed to see what life after Mom would be like. This job spelled optimism for Judi.

There was good news for Mom, too. Graduates of GARP were welcomed to join a day program to keep their good habits going and also offer respite for caregivers. We all thought it was perfect. But there was one hitch. Mom needed a driver to get there.

"I knew that job was too good to be true," Judi mourned. "I can't be the driver and do the contract, too."

"No problem," I said. "I'll drive. You have to take that job."

"But you have to get back to the Coast, don't you?" Mom and Judi said in unison.

"Nothing happening at home is more important than what is happening here. Count me in until Christmas. Then we can reassess." Mom protested, but weakly. I deserved my retirement. She hated me chasing around after her. What about Ed? Didn't my husband need me, too? Judi just said thanks. We would have more twin time. We felt silly talking about it, but both of us just felt more complete when we were together.

Now Mom had her new lease on life, Judi and I were determined that she wouldn't squander it. No way would we let Mom slip back into her old habits! We were in charge of her resurrection! We were bullies. In fact, the whole plan was a few shades of grey from outright elder abuse. "Operation

Maintain the Gain" we called it – OMG. We set out all the Activities of Daily Living on a long checklist, together with the specific things Mom said she wanted to do again. By assessing each item, yes or no each day, we could keep tabs on "progress." We assumed, without asking, that all this would motivate Mom.

As soon as Mom collapsed in her La-Z-Boy with a sigh of contentment, and her first rum and Coke in weeks was in her hands, we talked about OMG. Sure, we got Mom's input. But what choice did she have other than yes, yes, and yes again? Besides, she wanted to make this work for all of us just as much as we did. Perhaps Mom felt guilty that in spite of all our best efforts, she was still dwindling? Top of the OMG list were the bed and chair exercises that came home with her from GARP. They must be done daily. They must be done right. Then, she must get dressed every day, too. No more of this sitting around in a nightdress! Mom equivocated on this item. Why not wear her nightie? She liked it. We argued that it was giving up on life to not meet it head on every day in the right attire. Well, she said, the right attire didn't work for her because of all the fasteners. No worries! Judi and I trundled her in her wheelchair to the thrift store to stock up on frumpy but comfy clothes featuring Velcro and elastic. Personal hygiene? Tricky. How can daughters tell their mother that her breath stinks? Mom agreed it was a good idea to at least wash her face to get the glue out of her eyes and brush her teeth. Tending to this all by herself once a day went onto the OMG score sheet. There would be a fridge check. Were the Meals on Wheels dinners being eaten? We bought a jug for water, one quart a day, like it or not. Mom protested that coffee was just flavoured water, and so was rum with Coke.

We agreed. She agreed to take a full glass with her pills. And no more handfuls of pills when she remembered. She would take her medications as directed and when she was supposed to. The Lifeline pendant must stay around her neck, not sit by her bed tangled with her rosary. And every damn day, a walk. To the elevator and back. We were relentless. We were obsessively optimistic, too, and Mom said she'd be True Grit right along with us.

It started well enough. For at least a week all the check-marks were in all the right places, "Did you?" "Yes." But our visits shifted in tone. Instead of, "How are you feeling today, Mom?" our question was "What have you done?" Mom became sullen. Eventually she began to respond to the daily grilling with, "I failed that test, too, I guess." After a few weeks, we put the OMG checklist away. Mom rapidly slipped back to the way she had always been, the way she wanted to live. Judi and I recognized ourselves in the dance of co-dependence. The more we pushed, the less she did for herself.

Thank God…er…thank Source, for daycare! There was variety in those days and no goading was needed for Mom to participate. When she arrived at the daycare, she stretched out on her recliner in the row of other recliners, chatting to the old ladies and waiting for the next activity. She learned their names and stories. Some of those acquaintances became friends. Mom was freed from the biggest prison of her old age, her isolation.

"I want to wear my make-up again," Mom said one day. "Can you find my bag for me?" I rejoiced at this sign that classy Mom was still inside and wanted out. So I rummaged through her half-empty bottles and dried-out compacts and cracked nubs of bright red lipstick that would now be stark against her pale face, and found some blush, eye shadow and a lipstick that would work. "I'll get you fresh makeup," I said as I passed it over. "Do you want help?"

She didn't want help. When she emerged from the bathroom half an hour later, I gasped. The eye shadow had missed her eyelids and was a smudge above her eyebrows. Her blush was uneven and thick. Her lipstick was a slash between her upper lip and nostril. Of course she could not see this in the mirror! She was blind with macular degeneration in both eyes! How stupid of me. My clown mother smiled. "I'm ready." Mom's face beneath the mask looked delighted, coquettish even, as I helped her on with her coat. I gushed that she looked great, and she said thank you, she felt great, too. I excused myself, pleading a last minute trip to the bathroom. With the door closed, I phoned the nurse. "Please don't say anything," I whispered. "I told her she looks stunning and it would embarrass her."

"Good for Betty!" the nurse replied. She was delighted. This was a sign of her hope of better days ahead. We signed off, "OK, mum's the word."

The weeks passed quickly. But blue funk days took over from blue sky ones. The daycare doctor was worried. She said Mom spent too much time now sleeping. Her pain came roaring back as she moved less, and that new agony made her body stiffen more. It became a vicious circle of suffering. Along with that came the depression. Judi and I mourned. The Awakening had been a miracle, but it began to fade.

In November, I was surprised when Mom said she wanted to do her own Christmas baking. "Don't you start calling me manic now!" she admonished. "I just like making lots of cookies at Christmas." Of course, it was the hyper side of her bipolar reality but that didn't matter. Baking together would be fun. So we pored through her old recipe books, while she sipped rum and Cokes that were mostly Coke now, and found the ones most covered with grease spots from long-ago buttered hands. Those were the ones she wanted. She would bake a dozen for each of her helpers, and family too. This meant 600 cookies, 49 dozen give or take a few for tasting. She had a phalanx of specialists all interested in a different part of her body. Therapists kept the parts moving: physiotherapists, massage therapists and respiratory therapists. There were lifestyle helpers for manicures, pedicures, and haircuts. She had a woman who brought communion and a blind psychologist who sat with her every week to tease out her life story and help her face her wounds. John at the Safeway pharmacy said he felt he knew Mom personally, though he had only met her through her drug list. There were Goliath's care aides who came in and out. She had others that she paid for from her own resources. Most of all, there were all the nurses and friends at the daycare. That was just the beginning. Seven children, thirteen grandchildren, and an assortment of nephews and nieces all needed cookies. Mom told me to ask everyone in the family to recall their fondest Christmas-cookie memory. The final baking list included rolled sugar cookies in shapes of bells and trees, decorated with green and red sugar crystal sparkles. There were Rice Krispy squares, hairy eyeballs rolled in sweet shredded coconut, peanut-butter cookies squished into a design with a fork, macaroons and lots of rum balls. I filled the car several times with trunkfuls of ingredients and 49 festive cookie tins from the dollar store. When Mom was not at day care, we baked. The apartment was suffused with purpose and the smell of heated vanilla. My hunch about Mom's lack of spunk was accurate. She didn't have the energy, now that we had ingredients filling the dining room like some cottage industry. She could mix the dry ingredients but had no strength to stir the batters. She liked to sprinkle the decorations though, and enjoyed rolling the hairy eyeballs in coconut, remembering Matt as a little boy taking a whole batch to his room for a snack. She let me do the rest of the baking and sorting and washing up. When the stacks of tins were ready, Mom dictated a personal message of love or gratitude to go with each one. I guided her hand to scribble a signature. Then, with many stops for Christmas cheer, Judi and I delivered them all. I didn't want to see another cookie as long as I lived. But I had never enjoyed the Joy of Cooking as much as that marathon with Mom.

Though she insisted she was looking forward to Christmas on the Coast, I knew that wasn't true. Getting there was agony. Being there was comfortable enough but without her doctors around she felt vulnerable. Still, we had to press on with the plan. I was desperate now to be at home. Judi had plans to be away. Dad would be OK, but Mom needed care. She needed to be with me.

The airport nearest my home on The Coast was too small for a jetway, and used a scissor-lift platform to move food carts and the infirm off the plane. We arrived in a sleet storm, with a cold wet wind blowing off the ocean. I watched in helpless horror from behind the yellow "DO NOT CROSS" tape. Someone had forgotten Mom. "Sorry, Ma'am, you are not allowed to go there," the official said as I stormed past to rescue her, furious. She was huddled against the wind and whimpering. We got her home, moaning but assuring me that she was glad to be with us. Mom said she was comfortable by the fire and the big TV, looking out at the rain and the deep green forest. She struggled to be a cheerful guest. I did everything to make this the best holiday ever. My husband took many pictures of our intergenerational dream, with Nancy's family, too, gathered in the kitchen to make gourmet meals or relaxing in the living room with rum-laced eggnog we called moose milk. How could he record Mom's fatigue, her nausea, the throbbing back and stinging skin and the feeling she couldn't really put into words that doom was approaching? On Christmas Eve, we sat together and watched *It's a Wonderful Life*.

One night just after Christmas, Mom said her skin felt like it was burning in a fire. I couldn't see anything but believed her description as the worst pain she ever had. Desperate, my son Jamie and I went looking for any potion that might soothe her. We scoured central Vancouver Island for hundreds of miles through the dark, the windshield wipers hardly keeping up with the slashing rain. As we struggled from one all-night pharmacy to the next, I bared my soul to Jamie. I did not see how I could go on as a caregiver at a distance from my own home. It made me desperate to know that as bad as this night was, there was still no end in sight. I told him I feared for Judi, too. When I got to that part, I could not hold back my tears.

"Would Grandma accept me as her caregiver?" Jamie asked. At first, I could not believe what I was hearing. Could it be that someone else would be stepping up? My son was serious. As a physiotherapist, he said, he could work anywhere. He had no ties to the Coast right now. In fact, he was looking ahead to medical school and the University of Calgary was one of the possibilities. Sure, he could move to Calgary and live in that spare room she had. I asked if he would cook for her, since she had become tired of Meals on Wheels, and he said of course. I asked him if he minded helping her to the bathroom at night, and he said he walked with old ladies all the time in his job. I asked him if he would talk to her and be a companion, and he said Grandma was the most fascinating person he knew. When Mom heard, she was delighted. I guessed that she might see Judi and Janet as too much of a good thing. And of course Mom was no fool. She could see what a drag she was on us. Judi was not enthusiastic. Would Jamie be a boarder or a caregiver? What would happen on weekends? Could he keep to regular mealtimes and, really, did Jamie know how to cook? But Mom insisted it would all work out. "I just want to stay home," she repeated. "I want to stay out of an institution if I can." Judi knew her concerns were overridden by everyone else's optimism.

Jamie packed for Calgary.

11

Never-Ending Story

"Let the River Run."

My son arrived in January, shaken by his solo drive over the Continental Divide in a blizzard, and exhausted from the long trip. But he still regaled us with his stories of avalanches missed, warning lights blinking, and even a flat tire in the driving snowstorm. Mom glowed with pleasure to have her grandson moving in, and I was thrilled to return to the Coast and pick up the dropped threads of my life.

Judi still visited Mom often during the day, and Goliath's workers still came to help with homemaking and personal care as they did before. But now that Jamie filled the void on nights and weekends, Judi could make plans for herself for the first time in years. With this freedom came new patience. Mom and Judi delighted in their rediscovered mother and daughter companionship, and got back to Scrabble.

And Dad? While Mom's chances to remain independent at home had improved with Jamie's arrival, Dad's possibilities to stay in his seniors' residence with Martha suddenly evaporated. Martha found a lump in her stomach, and it had to be checked for cancer. She treated the biopsy as if it was the cancer operation, and said she was sure she was done for.

126

In a better situation Dad might have just needed a temporary solution while she recovered for a few days. But things between Martha and Dad were not going well. Martha was at the end of her tether, she said, and could not cope any longer with Fred. She did not have cancer, but we used the pretext of her illness to make Dad's move into assisted living. Martha bounced back and claimed she relished her solo life, fitting visits to Dad into her busy agenda.

At first Dad settled well into Shady Pines. He thought of the assisted-living facility as a resort. The nurses and aides were pretty. There were big TVs to watch and a little park to walk in and he liked the food better than Martha's soups. After a few months, though, Judi began to report that Dad was restless and morose. He missed his bride, he said, though he also admitted that she talked nonstop when she visited and he just turned off his hearing aids in self-defense. Judi thought he was lonely. But there was more. At the weekly happy hour, as they shared the one light beer Dad was allowed, Judi could see other residents shunning him. Dad called the other guests in the resort snooty. The administrator said Dad's dementia was progressing. In fact, the upper floors of Shady Pines, designed for cognitively intact residents, were not appropriate any longer for Dad. The administrator agreed that he had become isolated. "Elderly people often fear dementia in themselves and so avoid others who have it." Dad was like a wounded animal, rejected by his herd. We needed a solution. It arrived in the form of a studio apartment that came available in the memory care wing of Shady Pines. It was located in the basement behind doors that opened with a code punched into a key pad. This assured secure living for residents with dementia, and it was where Dad needed to be now. Still, we were sad for him. "At first he will find it strange, I think," said the administrator, "since he is stronger cognitively than most of the other residents." She sighed, "But that won't last long I'm afraid. Your father is failing fast."

My husband Ed and I took Dad on a weekend trip to Vancouver while Judi worked with Jamie, Chris and Linda to move Dad's stuff downstairs. We told Dad he would love his new digs because they cost half the price of what he was paying upstairs. Dad was happy. He had not lost his love of a bargain. The administrator was right; Dad did fail quickly. Just a few months after his moving downstairs we were driving with him past the seniors' lodge where Martha still lived. "I think I used to live somewhere around here." Dad wasn't upset about that. It was just a fact.

But Dad remained lonely. Calling from the Coast, I begged Jamie to visit his grandfather more often. Jamie responded as he always did. "Things are actually in pretty good shape around here, Mom. You know what I think? I think you and your twin worry way too much." I wasn't put off this time. Yes, but was he visiting his grandfather at all?

"I go when I can, Mom. But I can't and won't keep the pace of you and your twin." We changed the subject. Jamie told me about how he had taken Dad to an open house in the neighborhood mosque. He had been surprised, he said, at how tired and breathless Dad became, walking that half block.

"You walked?" I said. How could Jamie not know that Dad used a wheelchair now to go any distance? I held my tongue. Jamie assured me that once he'd caught his breath, his grandfather loved the place, especially the table of cookies. Jamie said he stuffed several into his pockets, for later. I smiled. Dad would never change. "Did he know where he was?"

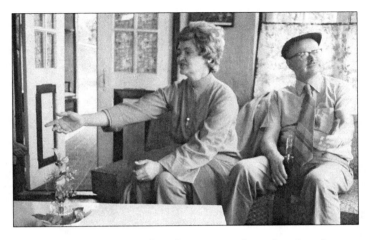

What dream were Fred and Betty reaching for that day in the early 70's when this picture was taken? Certainly it was not one of growing old together, even then. They divorced in the mid 80's after more than forty years of trying to make their marriage work.

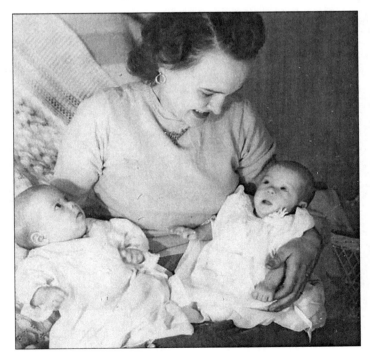

Judi and I were born six weeks prematurely in February, 1949. We were the second and third children of Fred and Betty Perry. Judi was six minutes older than me.

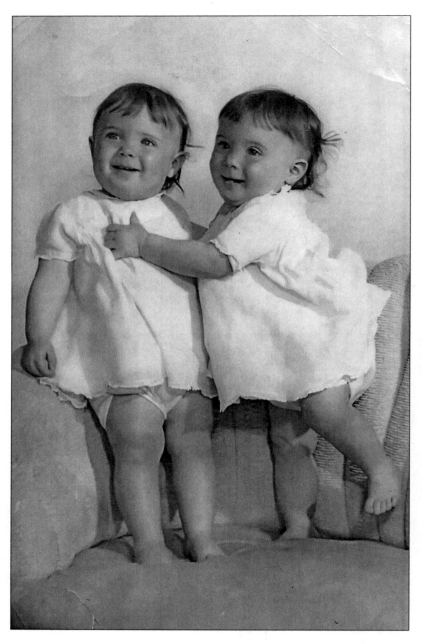

We have never stopped being each other's very best friend.

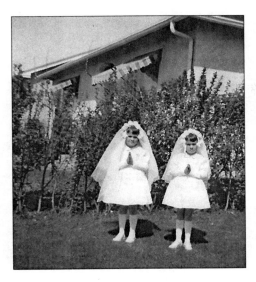

We twins grew up in a strongly
religious family of seven children,
in Calgary, Alberta, Canada.

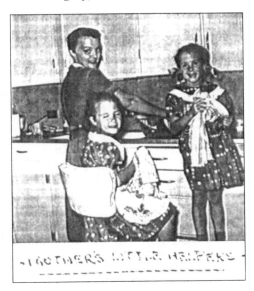

Judi and I were socialized to be
caregivers. In this old album, Dad
praised us as "Mother's Little
Helpers." Even by the age of seven
we both knew how to stand out in
the crowd of kids and perhaps even
get an extra dose of parental love.

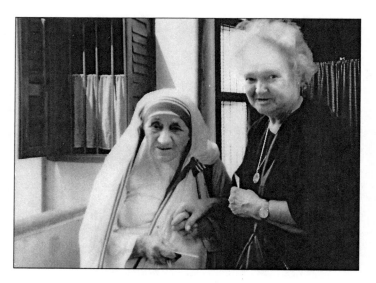

Mom set high standards of service. When she worked with Saint Teresa of Calcutta, Mom was the same age as Judi and I were as our own caregiving journey began at the dawn of the Millennium.

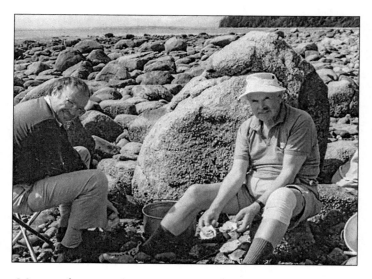

Mom volunteered in retirement, but Dad's dream was to live a vagabond life. He moved to a boathouse on a remote Gulf Island to live cheaply off the land. His eldest son watched with amusement as Dad showed him how he filched oysters from a private beach when the owners weren't looking. Dad was 73 and full of vigour.

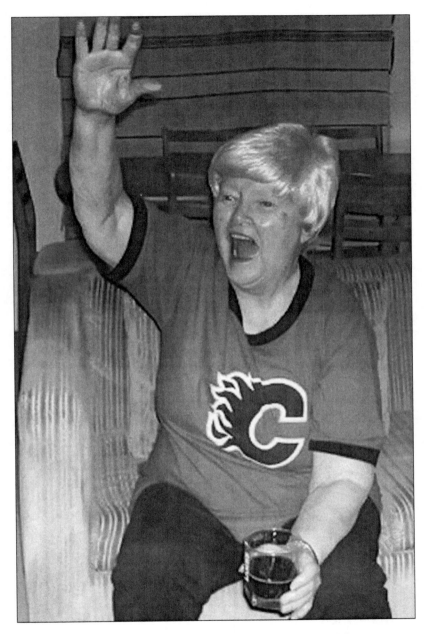

Though Mom's dwindling time began in 2000, she hid her growing infirmity as long as she could. Who would ever know from this picture of a raucous mother, celebrating a hockey win in her wig and team shirt, that she needed a wheel chair to move around, and hours of daily support to remain independent?

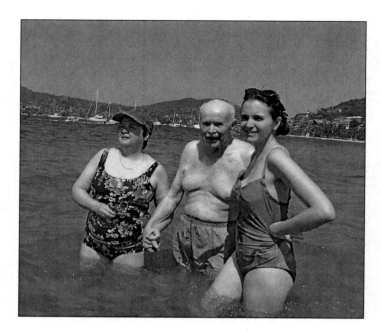

Dad needed help too. On this final holiday, my family took him to a beach in Mexico. He needed my daughter Fiona and me to help him take a dip in the Pacific.

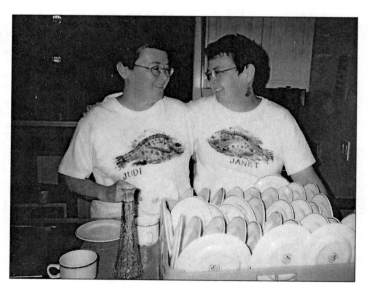

By the time Dad was 90, he was barely able to stay awake at the tea party we planned to celebrate his birthday. Judi and I were the twin team, and had hit our stride as caregivers.

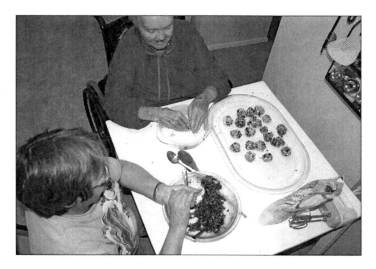

A favourite memory of Mom in the dwindling time was how we baked 49 dozen Christmas cookies to thank her caregiving team. Mom said she loved the feeling of being useful as much as she loved the smell of vanilla that infused her apartment for a month.

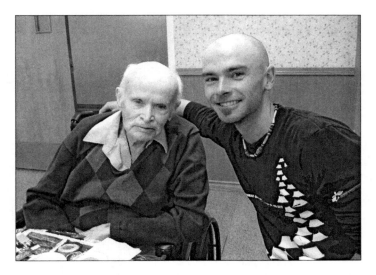

A favourite memory of Dad as he dwindled was how much he loved to talk about his budget funeral. Whether it was the sandwiches for his wake or the camping trip after his ashes were spread, no detail escaped Dads joyful attention. My son Jamie listened patiently each time his Grandpa rehashed the instructions for his send off.

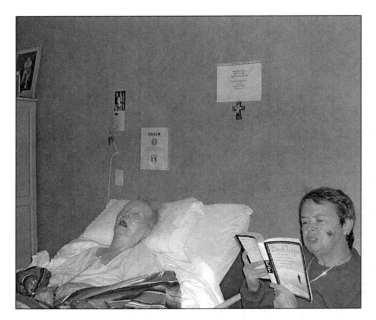

As Mom faded into helplessness, she entered another realm that was not often awareness. All we could do as caregivers was to sit with her, and read. On this Canada Day, the book was all about bad trips, and it seemed somehow suitable to the situation.

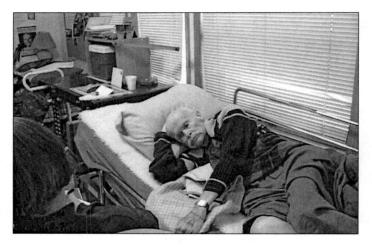

As Dad faded into helplessness, he just wanted his visitors to remind him of who they were. He would always respond with a gravelly-voiced "yup" when we told him how much he was loved.

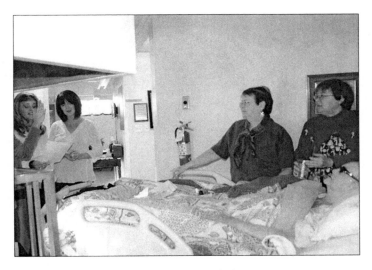

Spirit House was a hospice. It tended to Mom's now overwhelming needs, but also our emotional needs as family. We twins listened in exhaustion to carollers singing Silent Night. Was it unfortunate that Mom responded to the care by outliving her expected expiry date? She was moved again, and so the struggle for quality care went on for two more long years.

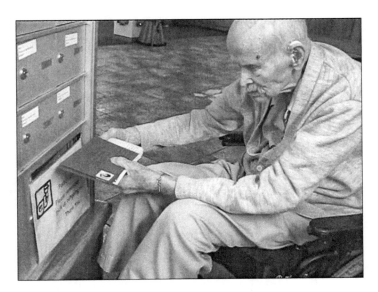

Dad mailed Christmas cards to his loved ones in December 2009. By the time they arrived at their destinations, he had died.

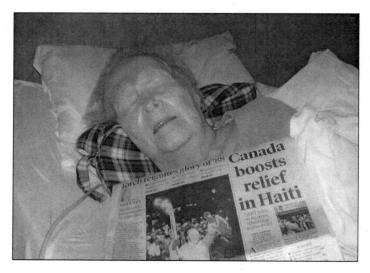

Mom seemed to be aware, even smile, when Judi read her
the news of the Olympic Torch Relay passing through Calgary in January 2010. How could we know, when Mom's
death seemed so near, that she would carry her own life
torch for another year before her time came to die?

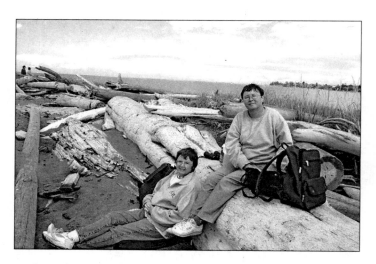

When the Parent Project was finally over, Judi and I were
exhausted. Still, we agreed that being caregivers for Mom
and Dad through their decade of dwindling was the hardest
job we ever loved.

"No way. He asked me who that nice man was, with a beard all dressed in white." We laughed about that, and I was relieved to step back from the tension with my son. "Grandpa's losing it pretty fast, isn't he, Mom?"

I agreed. "He might not have too many more months of even knowing who you are." Was I just giving Jamie a fact? Or was I trying to manipulate my son, make him feel guilty, perhaps goad him to visit Dad more often?

"Yah, I know." Jamie said, not catching my subtlety. Maybe just ignoring it. "But he was sure sharp telling me about his funeral arrangements." It was better to talk about Dad's foibles than his feebleness, and Jamie was right. Dad was obsessed with his death. We agreed Dad had done his research in his cognitively sharper times and that was serving him well now. He'd paid for a no-frills funeral, with no hearses, fancy chapels with deep carpet and hardwood walls, or people in pinstripe suits with long faces. He'd be cremated in a cardboard box and his ashes would be kept till his children could gather and spread them according to his precise directions. I told Jamie the story of how Dad had driven his congregation at the church to the brink of murder. He stalked the pastor at coffee hour always wanting to go over the arrangements one more time. She lost patience, and sent him to Sandy in the Ladies Guild. They were in charge of the post-funeral lunch, and this part was particularly important to Dad. He hated the tuna sandwiches they liked to serve and didn't want them anywhere near his funeral. "Egg salad sandwiches on brown bread with little bits of celery for crunch, please. Can you believe this guy?" Sandy complained to the pastor. "He doesn't get it that he's going to be dead!" Pastor Julie told Sandy to relax. It wasn't about sandwiches; it was about control. The poor man had so little of that in his life now, why not let him take charge of his funeral menu? Could the Ladies Guild humour him and promise not to serve tuna sandwiches?

If the pastor and Ladies Guild were challenged by Dad, Ben was overwhelmed. Pastor Julie had asked Ben to help with the elegy, a particularly worrisome element for Fred, she told him. Naïve about Dad, Ben had agreed with enthusiasm. It didn't last. Dad began to hound his elegist, even chasing him into the men's room after the Sunday service. Every week Dad had new thoughts or memories to add to the vignette pile.

Finally, Pastor Julie invited Dad to come with Judi and me to her office, "to review the plans." Dad was thrilled. Pastor Julie finally understood! His eyes glowing, we sat around Pastor Julie's desk. Dad worked through his dream of the perfect send off. Was the teenager who played the steel guitar in the choir still ready to play at the funeral? Would there be lots of cowboy hymns? Did she still have the money he had given her in a dozen envelopes to pay off everyone who would have their hand out, as he put it? Pastor Julie put both hands in the air, then covered her ears. "OK, stop it, Fred! That's enough!" She said there must be no more funeral talk. "God wants you to live now, so I want you to get on with that. Will you do that Fred? God will take care of your dying, and I assure you, you will be a satisfied customer at the end." So Dad turned the funeral file over to Judi, who put it away in the papers with all his research for trips long past.

Jamie liked that story. "Well, it's his next journey, after all," he said. He admitted he understood his grandfather better. I had one more anecdote. It was about ketchup. I had been having dinner with Dad at Shady Pines, and as always, he wanted to talk about his death. I asked if he was afraid of it, since it was such a focus. "Well," Dad said, slowly, the way he talked now, "actually being dead is no problem because after all…" he paused, "I will be dead." I waited. "It's the dying part that…" Dad didn't finish.

"What makes you worry about dying?" I probed. He didn't know exactly, but there were tears in his eyes. He was ready for some pain, of course, but that wasn't what bothered him. He admitted that he didn't want to be forgotten. I was overwhelmed with tenderness and took his hand in mine. Dad didn't pull away, as he would have through all my life with him. It felt so much like love to me, an intimacy I'd always longed for. Now I paused my story, swallowing hard. I knew Jamie was listening, not commenting, perhaps uncomfortable on the other end of the line. Was I was revealing too much of myself? I went on. I told Jamie that when the food arrived, Dad reached for the ketchup as he always did, and squirted an enormous glob over his meat loaf. When he was done, I picked up the bottle. "Dad, whenever I see one of these, I will always think of you." I couldn't go on. A sob seemed to be holding back my words. Jamie understood. He agreed that a ketchup bottle was a great way to remember Dad when he was gone. "That's a great story, Mom, thanks for sharing."

Jamie had promised to cook regular meals for Mom, and he kept his commitment. What I didn't realize at first, though, was that he knew only one recipe. It was for a one-pot rice-based meal, with mounds of vegetables, in a choice of four varieties of sauces that came in jars. He called all his food "Chicken Vindaloo." Though Mom said she loved his way with curry, she admitted to me that she had lost her taste for spice. That was not the biggest problem, though. It was his wish that she eat with him, sitting at the table. Before Jamie arrived, Mom had come to like having dinner served to her on a tray in her La-Z-Boy. While she ate, she watched the news hour on CNN. Sitting on the stiff-backed chair hurt her back.

"I don't want to feed you in your recliner," Jamie insisted. "You need to move." Mom tried to cooperate at first, lurching from the recliner to the table, gripping the back of the sofa and the wall. She even smacked her lips at first, praising Jamie for his cooking prowess. Perhaps Jamie didn't notice. Perhaps Jamie didn't care. But when Mom began to leave most of the Chicken Vindaloo on her plate, Judi became concerned. Night after night, at the tuck-in visit, Mom said she felt a little peckish and asked for a poached egg maybe, or a bowl of cream of chicken soup or a grilled cheese sandwich, just to fill the holes in her stomach, she said. Judi began to bring an extra plate of the dinner she had made for Tom, and reheat it as a bedtime snack for Mom. Judi claimed this was Jamie's failure. Jamie called it Judi's over-performing. I tried not to think about it at all.

The coffee war made Chicken Vindaloo seem like a minor skirmish. Mom loved her morning coffee, brought to her in her recliner while she listened to CNN. To Jamie, her love of this routine was another opportunity for forcing her to get up and move. Just walking to the kitchen was something, at least. So, each morning, Jamie got the coffee ready to brew. As he kissed his grandmother good-bye on his way to work, he reminded her that everything was ready to go when she wanted her coffee and all she needed to do was push the button. He reminded her that this was an Activity of Daily Living, and anyway, fresh coffee was a much better start to her day than coffee sitting in the pot too long. Mom promised and said she understood about the importance of movement. Mid-morning, when Judi arrived to see Mom sitting in her recliner and hear that she had not had coffee yet, she brewed it and brought it to her chair. As she took the coffee, Mom assured Judi that she was a good daughter. Jamie suggested that she was an enabler.

Judi began to admit it. She was miffed with my son. I saw Mom playing them off against each other. Could she be doing this on purpose? What a fine line it was, I thought, between fostering dependence and being supportive! Judi and Jamie both had it wrong, I mused, in their extremes. But balance was elusive. Still, in this Cold War, I stood with Judi.

My brother Chris and his wife Linda moved to Calgary. At first Judi was delighted. Reinforcements! They were full of good intentions when they arrived. Mom loved their daily visits. But life got in the way as Chris and Linda settled in. They bought a house at the far edge of Calgary, an hour's drive in traffic to Hull Estates. They ran a business in a suburban mall, too. It had killer hours of operation that sucked up any spare time. And then, Judi said, there was the puppy. She pouted, and Chris pushed back. "We've got a life, you know," he said. "Give me any job I can do from my desk at home and when I have time, I'll do it gladly." We brainstormed over the phone and email. Was there such a job? I suggested that Chris could take over Martha management, calling her from time to time and overseeing the financial tug of war as Martha looked for more money to run her life as wife at a distance. Chris said he could do that fine and was willing to play hard ball with her if he needed to. Now Judi could say to Martha, "You need to talk about that with Chris." The arrangement worked well. But there was still one problem.

Every time that Chris and Linda arrived for a drive-by visit, Mom gushed with gratitude. Judi was miffed. She said she felt like oxygen. Essential, but taken for granted. It was a bitter truth. Absence made Mom's heart grow fonder. My visits, and those of my siblings, were great events. I reminded Mom and Dad every time I spoke to them how fortunate they were to have Judi, and they always agreed. But still her presence was accepted as nothing special.

Every six months, Goliath sent a social worker to check on Mom. Fragile elders were encouraged to stay in their homes, and no one wanted that more than Mom. But living independently was only possible as long as they could still accomplish the Activities of Daily Living. So the visit was also a test. Judi told me how the social worker asked Judi to leave her alone with Mom, and how she hovered in the kitchen to eavesdrop. She went through the list of questions and Mom's answers while I listened, trying not to laugh.

"Can you dress yourself?"

"Yes, every morning as soon as I am up. I've decided not to wear my bra, though, can't reach the hooks."

"Very good," the social worker said. "Do you wash your face and brush your teeth?"

"Oh yes. But I need a bath lift. Is there any chance I can get one of those?"

"Can you prepare food and do you eat three nutritious meals a day?"

"I never miss a meal. Canada Food Rules, you know!" I laughed and wondered if Mom might be pulling the social worker's leg.

Judi admitted she wasn't sure. She went on.

"Can you use the telephone?"

"What a silly question! Of course I keep in touch with all my children and my friends every day."

"Do you walk?" The social worker was pleased with this one, Judi said.

"Well, not so much. I'm in constant pain, you know. But I do get downstairs every day to get my mail. I do my laundry, I buy groceries."

It was hilarious, but at the same time, it was no joke. Did Mom mention you, I wondered. Judi's voice told me she was angry now.

"My daughter visits from time to time," Mom told the social worker.

"Time to time. Where does she get the nerve to say you help from time to time?" I was irritated. Judi was perplexed. What was true for Mom and what was her active fibbing and what was just her wishful thinking? The social worker had praised Mom. She was doing so much better than most of her clientele. It was proof of the success of a programs like GARP and the daycare. But there was a catch. She no longer qualified for the same level of assistance from Community Home Support because she was managing too well.

Judi said she confronted Mom about this interview. Less help from Goliath meant more jobs right back on her plate. Mom just sniffed. Judi could choose how much to help. But if no more strangers came to feed her cold soup or slather cream on her feet she'd be A-OK with that. "Let's just let the river run," she said. There was nothing left to say, she said.

I wouldn't be put off, though. "Why, Mom," I asked when I called her later that day, "did you tell the social worker all those fibs?" I could hear Mom's tone turn icy. "You girls just don't get it. I know I could do all the things she asked. I just don't feel like it. Anyway, isn't it my business?" I didn't want an argument. Her fear about losing independence made this a touchy subject.

At her next six-month visit from the social worker, though, Mom answered honestly. The social worker was shocked. How could Mom have got so much worse so fast? She couldn't perform any of the ADLs that she had accomplished so easily just months before. She needed to get on a waiting list for long-term care, pronto. The social worker explained that if Mom wound up in hospital, as she surely would sooner rather than later at the rate she was declining, she would have to take the first bed available in long-term care. It might be far away. It would probably be less suitable. The high-performing places were popular and had long waiting lists. The social worker left Judi with the forms. "Don't delay this any longer."

This plunged Mom into a blue funk. "You girls decide what to do," she commanded in a flat voice. "I don't care where I wind up." She told Judi to scram and to close the curtains and turn off the TV. "Find me a place in Timbuktu."

Judi whimpered. She raged. She said we needed to look at all the nursing homes in Calgary and make a choice: one, two or three. Would I come out and help? We were all business when I arrived, and over a beer or two developed a checklist of must-have and nice-to-have factors for Mom's nursing home. Top priority for me was a place close by. Calgary's sprawl meant a driving challenge at the best of times. Judi hated navigating through heavy traffic, and she would still be visiting Dad. Could we request Shady Pines, I wondered? Judi said Mom nixed that right away. There was no way that she would risk ever having visits from Dad.

Inconvenient or not to visitors, she must be in her own long-term-care centre. We eliminated Shady Pines. Judi said she wanted a place where family would be part of the care team, not put up with or worked around. There were many places that were not family friendly. Mom would also need a room of her own. Those talking books were loud and headphones were out of the question. They had already caused ear ulcers. There didn't need to be a lot of recreation in the perfect place, but spiritual care was essential. People to talk to would be an asset but we knew that was tricky. Mom needed to engage at a high level of conversation, and that was hard to find among the very old. Judi laughed as she pointed out that Mom's only body part still working reliably well was her brain. And her taste buds sometimes. Fancy menus didn't matter much because we would still be bringing in the treats like scallops and lobster, no matter where she landed.

We went from facility to facility over two long weeks. Some were brand new, and some were heritage buildings. Some had been carefully decorated inside and out, others looked shabby. We timed our tours to late morning or afternoon, when residents would be active in a place with a good ambience, or snoring in their beds if the atmosphere was wrong. Each tour made me feel sadder. What a way to end up a full life! We kept reminding ourselves that we were not putting Mom away. If the place was not perfect, we would not accept it.

One facility seemed just right. It was an easy drive for both Judi and Chris, who would be the only regular visitors Mom could expect eventually. The director seemed knowledgeable about the residents and downright chatty, in fact. Her good cheer seemed authentic. There were single rooms, and even a garden with areas for visiting. Religious services happened daily in a purpose-built chapel. The dining room had tables covered in plastic linen and even LED-light candles. The activity board showed that the facility offered meaningful recreation: scrapbooking, storytelling and readers coming from the library for a book club. Kindergarten children came to visit. Judi and I were melting with relief. We had found the right place!

"We think it is important for our residents to see lots of animals around," the director explained as a Great Dane walked by tugging on its leash. "We have lots of visitor doggies, ferrets, and even a Shetland pony once in a while." She was proud of this asset. "Animals have such a calming energy, don't you think?" Judi jabbed me and pointed. A large black cat crouched on the nurse's station, hissing with its tail in the air. "Oh yes! And we do have several kitties. Our residents love them. We give them the run of the place. Animals seem to just know who is needy, don't you agree?" We crossed Greenfields off the list. Mom hated cats.

We also crossed off the facility where the director insisted residents with dementia should be mixed in with the residents who had, as she put it, "all their marbles." She confided that anyone who arrived cognitively intact wouldn't stay that way long. While Dad had shown us that was true, it felt strikingly disrespectful. Mom's marbles must be cherished.

We joined a group tour in a newly-opened facility, and were impressed by the amenities. There were soaker tubs, huge TV screens, and in the activity room there was a large fireplace with a facing of river rocks. Then I heard a wail, "Help me, help me, someone help me!" The director didn't flinch. Farther down the hall someone else in a wheelchair reached out to grab my arm saying, "Get me out of here." A cacophony of call bells punctuated the director's smooth presentation. She ignored all of it. Unsettled, I asked about all this. There was a staff shortage, she admitted and, anyway, staff found that if they didn't give into these plays for attention, they would stop. That place went off the list.

After each tour Judi and I found a pub to debrief. We became more morose as the days went on. Poor Mom! We decided to just share our research with her and leave the decision in her hands, where it belonged.

I could tell she was not paying attention as Judi presented the assets and liabilities of each place. "So, what do you think?" I asked when Judi was done.

"What about Lacombe? I told you I wanted Lacombe." We were ready for this objection. Though it was the one Catholic Church-run facility in Calgary, it took more than an hour to drive door to door, even on a good day. Judi and I had agreed it was impossible. "But I want Lacombe," Mom repeated.

"You need to give three choices." I was exasperated.

"No I don't. I will only go to one nursing home and that's Lacombe and that's final." I heard Mom's stubborn voice. "Listen here, kiddos. These are my choices. One: Lacombe. Two: Lacombe. Three: Lacombe. Now go away. I want to be alone." She asked that we close the curtains and turn off the lights and the TV. We knew we had failed.

Life dragged on through the cold Calgary winter. As Judi often said now, "Let the river run." She cared for Mom as she had in the days before Jamie's arrival. His door stayed shut in the evenings now. He was studying intensively for a bid to get into medical school and said that organic chemistry was a monster of a challenge. When I pressed him to talk about how things were going, he admitted this was not the situation he expected when he came to live with his Grandma. "It's a never-ending story, all this need, all the time, isn't it?" he said.

12

Good Twin, Bad Twin

"It was you who poisoned the water!"

J amie and Judi reached an accord. I was a calming influ-
ence, I hoped, on both of them. Judi vented when there
was a clash between her work for pay and her work for love.
Jamie vented when his expectations of himself got out of
balance with the time he really had, or when Judi's demands,
as he saw them, went over the top. His frustrations came out
indirectly, as comments and observations, never complaints.
Once he said we twins were bikers pedaling furiously in 16th
gear. I Googled that to find it meant we were working hard
but getting nowhere, with the implication we were over-func-
tioning and, well, just being stupid. I was miffed, but Jamie
was right. Caregiving meant spinning in high gear. It was
unrelenting effort for not much progress.

Mom and Dad dwindled differently. Mom's slide was
physical, but her mind stayed strong. Dad kept more physical
resources, at least enough to toddle around his immediate
environment, but his mind was slipping away.

I stayed in daily touch with Judi. I had a template on my
cell phone with the message, "How is she?" and Judi replied by
number. A terrible day was a 1, and then I phoned to talk. A

great one was 5, and I went about my business feeling content. Mom's reality had settled to about a 3.

That Easter I visited Mexico. I was anxious about leaving the country, even for two weeks, but it was clear to me that my husband needed me as much of me as Judi did. We had a good time together, and as long as the number was 3 in the daily text, I relaxed. With a few days left to go in our getaway though, there was a cryptic message on my cell phone instead of the number. "Blisters forming. Maybe shingles. Call me." My finger trembled as I punched in Judi's number. I heard her all-business voice which told me she was frightened. Mom had a blistering rash and more bumps were popping up every few minutes. The staff at the daycare noticed it first when Mom felt something very wrong with her arm and over her breasts. The doctor said shingles and sent her home. When the blisters filled with fluid, Judi sent the text. So far away, there was little I could do but listen and share her fears. But the blisters were not the biggest problem. The most worrisome thing about Mom was her manner. She was hard to wake, and when she did, wow! Judi said she stared with blank eyes and her fingers picked at imaginary flies in the air. I rerouted my ticket to go to Calgary, rather than home to the Coast. My husband muttered, "Here we go again, when will it ever end?" I had no answer for him. "What does Doc Nan say?" I texted Judi. She replied right away.

"Take her to Emergency."

"Then do it!" I shouted my reply in capital letters.

There was one final text from Judi as I boarded my fourth and final flight to get to Calgary. "Hurry." My brother Chris was waiting to meet me. "Judi can't leave Mom," he said as he enveloped me in a hug and took my bag. Usually unflappable, I could see that Chris was jangled now. "Mom is just blotto," he said. "I've never seen anything like it." We drove a little too fast down the Deerfoot freeway, Chris weaving in and out of traffic. "You are the power team," he began, and then gripping the steering wheel added, "but we'll need to put her away now, like it or not. This can't go on."

"Put her away?" He stiffened at my tone. We were silent. He stared at the road. I studied my hands. There was nothing I could say. I was not going to talk about putting Mom away.

At Mom's apartment I took one deep breath in and let it out, trying to be calm, and then opened the door. "Hi Mom! I'm back from Mexico!" I chirped. She had no reaction.

"See what I mean?" Chris whispered. "She's really out of it, worse actually than when I left to get you at the airport."

Mom's head snapped up. "Hi, Mom!" I tried again. "It's me, Janet."

She peered at me, her eyes flashing flint now, and then she snapped, "Get out of here!" My gut clenched. Mom looked at Judi and looked back at me. She pointed a trembling finger in my direction. I could see the blisters on her arm. "Bad twin! Bad! Go away!" I shivered in panic but tried to smile. "Don't you look at me with that twisty grin! I know you poisoned the water!"

"Let's call 911," was all I could say. "Why have you waited so long?" If they were frozen in indecision, boiled frogs still paddling around, I was galvanized to act. "I'm calling for an ambulance right now."

For the third time in as many months, paramedics rolled Mom down the hall on a squeaky gurney, drawing the neighbours to their doors shaking their heads and muttering, "Good luck." At the hospital the triage nurse said Mom was having a psychotic episode and asked Judi if she had an overdose. We didn't know. "Of course not," Judi said, haughty.

"She needs restraints," the nurse replied.

"No. We will stay with her." My advocate's helmet once again made me forceful. I would not allow straps over her flaming sore skin. Mom's aggression was only verbal. It was only directed at me. Judi could hold her hand and I could hide behind the curtain. "We will keep the sides up," I said, "that's plenty. She poses no danger."

The nurse accepted that. "Just don't leave her alone."

Yell and act crazy all you can, Mom, I thought. Be the squeakiest wheel in the place. We were Emergency Room experts. We knew quiet people, humble people, compliant people and, most of all, old people with daughters, could wait for many hours. Hysterics helped get to the head of the line. Chris said he was tired and he had to work in the morning. With me there, the twin team was invincible. He could leave. Did we need him, too, in the crowded space? I tried to find empathy for my tired brother. I didn't want to pick a fight with him. Could he not see that we needed him, I wondered? "Off you go, Chris," I said, managing an insipid smile. "Of course we can manage." As soon as he was gone, I called Jamie and asked him to come. We needed backup.

An intern pulled back the curtain. "What have we here?" he asked, but didn't wait for an explanation. "I'll just give her something to calm her down." Mom still picked at invisible flies that seemed to buzz around her head. She still didn't want me in her sight. But she relaxed, and so did we. Sometime later, another doctor arrived and introduced himself as that shift's attending physician. His name was Dr. Cook. "Are you twins?" I said I was the bad twin and told him about the poisoned water.

"Poor lady, I'm guessing meningitis. It can cause paranoia. I need an X-ray and a sample of spinal fluid. Do either of you have a power of attorney for personal care? She can't speak for herself." Judi pulled out the document from Mom's Emergency Room kit bag. Dr. Cook was impressed. "I wish all the people who came in here were so on the ball as you," he said. "Let me see."

"We've been through this rigmarole plenty of times before," Judi said. "Emergency Room management is part of our expertise."

"Mine too," Dr. Cook replied with a smile. "So, we're a team." I liked the guy. Being respected that way was unusual and it felt good. Judi passed over Mom's list of medications too. "She could not have had an overdose. Her meds are all in bubble packages."

Mom was awake again and screamed as she was wheeled down the hall, with Judi beside her and gripping her hand, mumbling prayers. Getting these tests done would be a challenge. I was glad I was not invited.

"It's not meningitis," Dr. Cook said when the results came back hours later. "That's the good news. But there is definitely something amiss somewhere. She needs to be admitted so we can figure it out." Then he smiled and looked at me. "By the way," he said, "your mother says I've poisoned the water, too." He agreed that the psychosis was an unpleasant symptom for everyone, but not something that was hurting her. But something needed to be figured out, and that's why she needed to be in the hospital for a time. I stammered my thanks, and relief.

The doctor was right. A few days later Mom could not imagine calling me a bad twin and laughed out loud about the poisoned water. She seemed to have more energy than I had seen for months. I told her about Mexico and she told me about hospital life. The blisters were oozing sores now, beginning to heal, the nurses said. Mom seemed to be on the mend for now.

Ten days after her admission, a stranger in a lab coat bustled into Mom's room and introduced himself as the dermatologist on call. He was trailed by a group of young men and women with stethoscopes around their necks, and clipboards. The doctor summarized 'the case' as he splashed water over his hands and then asked Mom, "What seems to be the problem?" He didn't wait for an answer, though, but poked at one or two of her lesions and squinted at her chart. To his groupies he said, "It is Bullous pemphigoid, an autoimmune condition." He poked some more and told the students that the usual treatment for this malady, prednisone, was not indicated in someone so old and frail. Therefore, they would do nothing beyond preventing infection. The specialist then scribbled a sentence or two on Mom's chart, and turned to leave, already asking a student for a rundown on the next patient. I barred the door, my advocate's helmet firmly fixed on my head, my slingshot loaded.

"Wait a minute!" I said, "We need more information than that! What is this thing you are talking about, this Bullous pemphigoid? How did she get it? Will it happen again? Will it get worse? What can we do to prevent it? To treat it?" The doctor was flustered. He glanced at his watch, and glared at me, and rattled off staccato answers. "Bullous pemphigoid is very rare. It is an autoimmune condition. Your mother's body is attacking itself for some reason I don't know. It might never come back or keep coming back, I don't know that, either. As for treatment, there are ointments to soothe the lesions and infection must be prevented. If people die of Bullous pemphigoid, it is because of infection. He turned back to face Mom, exhorting her to keep her skin squeaky clean at all times.

"Did you say there is no cure?" I pressed again. He was impatient now.

"No treatment for her." Then he was gone.

I raced to the nearest patient-support computer kiosk to consult WebMD. Everything the specialist said was right. Bullous pemphigoid was going to be a game-changer for Mom and us. But what about the blood test to confirm that this was really the problem, or not? What if it was just an allergic reaction to one of her many meds? Or a virus maybe? Wasn't it crucial to know if this was really Bullous pemphigoid? If Mom was going to have this happen again, then she would need more care than she could get at home. I began to stalk the hospitalist, seeking answers. I caught up with him the next morning at the elevator, a coffee in his hand, and told him what was at stake for Mom. We needed to be sure of this diagnosis. We needed the blood test done. "I'll look at her chart when I get some time. Now excuse me, I must be on my way." For the rest of the day, I raged at the offhanded way that the doctors handled this life-altering information. Jamie said he understood, but he was realistic, too. "Think about it, Mom," he said, "you know that Grandma will have to go to a nursing home sooner or later. Well, perhaps this means the time has come. Isn't it time to just give in and move on?"

Was I the boiled frog now, too? I wondered. Why was putting Mom into long-term care so hard for me to accept? Part of my challenge with all this was that Mom changed every day. One day she was in a stupor. The next she was hyper and full of energy. When it was blotto Mom, long-term care was a no-brainer decision. But wide-awake Mom would hate to be put away. These swings in her condition confused everyone, including Goliath's transition administrator. She was the person responsible for the big decision about long-term care. She couldn't make up her mind about what to do. She got off her fence, though, the day she came by to get some signatures and found Mom staring out the window. Could she see the tanks rolling down the Glenmore trail? They were Chinese invaders, didn't she know? And what about that ship in Glenmore Reservoir? It was full of feces, didn't she know? And by the way, did she know the water was poisoned and it was the bad twin who did it? There was no doubt. Long term care had to be. The administrator was frank, though. Mom would have to accept the first available bed in a long-term-care centre prepared to take her. She might need to wait quite a while in hospital for such a bed. There was a backlog. Judi grimly set about supporting Mom through what challenges lay ahead. I was relieved to leave for the Coast, promising to return as soon as Mom got a bed somewhere.

To keep busy, I worked on a briefing book. It would tell the story of Betty Perry and help her be known to the people who would be caring for her. It went through many versions as I came to terms with my conflicted emotions. The first version told the story of Betty Perry as strong and intelligent, well read, spiritual, but also a complicated woman. I hoped her resume, starting from birth, would prove to her caregivers that she was a woman of real consequence, deserving of the highest respect. In the next version, I focused on the qualities that would make Mom an easy person to care for. She was patient and kind and could endure. Her Catholic faith was profound. She had a sense of humour. Now I found myself writing and ripping, unsure now of what I really meant to convey about her personality. It depended on the day, didn't it? Finally, I just collected family pictures and introduced all of my siblings, Mom's kids, adding their kids' names and where they all lived and their jobs, and I knew this was not helpful. But at least with this version the staff at wherever Mom landed would know how much she was loved and supported by her large family. And the rest of it? They would have to figure it out themselves. The book might trigger a conversation or two, I hoped.

A bed became available. River Vista Manor was not on our list. Judi took a tour. She said the building was old and shabby. It was not so far from Hull Estates but hard to get to in rush hour. Four residents shared a bathroom and all the rooms had two occupants. Mom could get on a waiting list for a single room, Judi said, but the Director held out little hope for that. Mom's tiny space would be by a window, though, looking out on a garden of potted plants that the Director called 'The Atrium'. I knew Judi was trying hard to be upbeat but her voice shook as she described the place. She noticed a smell of mold in the Atrium, from overwatered plants perhaps. The visiting area was meant to have the feel of a tropical garden, with chairs around tables and colorful umbrellas. There weren't enough of them. Judi wanted my advice.

"Take the spot," I said. "Mom needs to move on. We all have to move on." I told her I was on my way to help with the transition.

Judi and Chris wrestled Mom's La-Z-Boy into the corner. Chris complained it took all the space but Judi insisted Mom would need a familiar place to sit. River Vista Manor's furniture was uncomfortable-looking and upholstered in plastic. Chris said she was the boss, and plunked the television set on the chipped wooden dresser as she directed. Then Judi went to the electronics store and bought yards of wires to rig Mom's headphones to the television, up to the ceiling and along the rail of the stained privacy curtain. Chris said that Ella, her roommate, was stone deaf and wouldn't hear CNN blasting anyway. But Judi was on a mission to make things perfect for Mom in this sad little cubbyhole where she was coming to live.

"I did my best," Judi murmured as I came off the plane. We collapsed into each other's arms and cried. Then we blotted our tears with a shared tissue. This was not a good time to get maudlin. There was never any time for public shows of defeat. I got my suitcase off the baggage carousel and by the time we were in the car, both of us had found our optimistic twin-team mode again. Long-term care was going to be a big adjustment for all of us. But at least we could be daughters instead of the little nurses now. Was putting Mom on the toilet and helping her wash her face and cleaning up after her accidents really the best use of Judi's time? Was it the best way to show her love?

"God is in charge," Judi said this over and over, her mantra. But this time we said it in unison. How could we read each other's minds? Finish each other's sentences? Express the very same thought in the same instant? It was something really deep about being twins. We loved it.

The traffic was snarled. As we waited, Judi complained about River Vista Manor. Though Mom had been there less than two days, Judi was already locking horns with the

Director. "What a piece of work she is!" Judi grumbled. While we crept along, she rattled off the rules she'd stumbled over so far by breaking them. Which stairwell could visitors use? Which bathroom? Where could visitors go for private visits? What parts of River Vista Manor were out of bounds? What hours could she visit? She told me there was a sign-in and sign-out rule. There was no outside food allowed without checking first with someone, she wasn't sure who. There would be no heaters brought in, even if Mom was cold, and no fans to cool her if she got hot. If the ventilation was bad in River Vista Manor, the wiring was far worse, Judi said. And the plumbing! There were creaks and cracks as toilets flushed and water ran hot and suddenly cold in the taps.

As Judi talked, a heaviness settled around my heart. Mom would need me more than ever to be her advocate at a distance, getting the information from Judi and making a stink if I needed to. Judi would need to be careful about complaining directly. But she would be the monitor of Mom's care. "They say that safety of the residents is their primary concern," Judi scoffed. We were turning the last corner toward River Vista Manor. "My ass! It's covering the ass of River Vista Manor staff that the rules are about. Patient-centred care? What bullshit!"

I was prepared for the worst. But Judi had also found assets at River Vista Manor, and they were people. I met one as I arrived, a middle-aged man named Lorne. He was the charge nurse. "Are you twins?" he asked, looking back and forth between Judi and me. As we went to Mom's room down the dingy hall, she said he had a great sense of humour and was tender with Mom. Lorne liked her spunk, she said, though Judi wondered what he could have seen of that so far.

Mom sure didn't show spunk with her! Dr. Lindquist was also solid gold, Judi reported. He was the resident geriatrician, though he wasn't really resident. Dr. Lindquist had hundreds of patients in long-term-care centres all over town, but he was amazing. He still seemed familiar with Mom's situation, and Judi said there was a good vibe between them.

I was shocked by Mom's room. Her space. I breathed for calm. "This place seems lovely," I lied as I bounced up to Mom and kissed her cheek. "You've lucked out to wind up here." Mom smiled wanly. She knew the game. It was called "make the best of it" and there was one motto: "God is in charge."

The grey metal hospital bed squeezed beside Mom's recliner, with a TV table for her gear and one folding chair for a visitor, brought in from near the door. Judi was right. I noticed the smell of the Atrium right away. The window was the only natural light in the room, and as the day was cloudy the lights needed to be turned on. Mom's portrait as a beautiful young nurse hung over her bed, gazing into her future and at the caregivers below. It was Judi's strategy, like my briefing book. We both wanted everyone to see a woman of consequence inside the wizened patient, to feel compassion for her. Judi had hung the portrait of Jesus as a young boy over the TV, in Mom's line of vision if she looked sideways at it, past the blot of her Macular Degeneration. It was Mom's favorite picture.

Ella was nice. She was deaf, though, and we had to shout to be heard. Ella was sure that River Vista Manor was full of thieves who went through her drawers at night. She promised to stay awake and guard Mom's stuff. Roommates had to stick together, she said in her crackly voice. The Director insisted residents always exaggerated these things. Still, she acknowledged that there were wanderers who might well think stuff belonging to others was theirs. River Vista Manor mixed the cognitively intact, that demeaning medical term, with residents in dementia. "Most residents are not that well oriented," Lorne said, "and, yes, some residents do go in and out of doors. The rules say they must not be closed, especially at night for safety reasons." He added that so far none of the residents were violent. "Panty raids are possible, but no manslaughter yet, thank God." He smiled. I did not.

I found that the saddest part of River Vista Manor was the dining room. The residents sat at Formica tables and waited for the food to be served from large trolleys in the middle of the room. The fluorescent lights buzzed. Eating off a tray in her recliner, the way she took her meals at home once Jamie had given up trying to change that, was not allowed here. We pushed Mom in her wheelchair to the assigned table, where three other women ignored our presence. They were deep in a silent conversation that they conducted by waving stuffed animal toys. Mom said she would get used to it, even find this slapstick funny. Judi told me in a whisper that after the first night of this, she had begged the Director to sit Mom at another table. There was one, with three women whom Judi observed having a real conversation, not staring blankly like everyone else was doing. It was impossible, though. The Director said that those ladies didn't want anyone else to join their group. And that was that. Mom's isolation began the first day.

The lack of any place to pray was the toughest pill for Judi to swallow. She had rooted out the plywood cross from behind a stack of chairs in the activity room and asked about it. The Director said she didn't know when or if there were religious services. It depended on who came to visit. "Religion isn't important to the residents here," the Director assured Judi.

"Well it is to one," Judi retorted, angry.

"Don't stay, girls," Mom said after my first dreadful dinner. "I need to get used to it. I actually want to get used to it. I'm sure I can get used to it. God is in charge. Go." She fumbled for her purse to pay us back for the $10 each that our dinner with her had cost. "Where's my wallet?" she said in alarm. Judi had to admit she had taken it away for safe-keeping. It was Mom's first personal indignity.

The front door was locked. I rattled it in frustration. "Did you sign out?" A nasal voice from behind what seemed like bullet-proof glass told us the code. The lockup protected wanderers, the voice said. But it confirmed my impression of River Vista Manor. The place was a prison. As we walked to the car, I wiped my tears while Judi swore and said we should have held out for a more suitable place. But we decided that we should let the river run for a while, and be patient. Things would look better once our shock wore off and we were used to the new routines.

Mom slept day and night. Dr. Lindquist assured us this was a normal first reaction of residents entering long-term care. Dissembling was easier than fury, or despair. He was right. I went home to the Coast for a while. When I returned on my next visit a few weeks later, to back up Judi going on a business trip, I found Mom sitting in her La-Z-Boy, saying she loved the view of the Atrium, and was delighted to see me. "Let's go for a walk by the river." I was overjoyed as I pushed her in her wheelchair through the June breezes along the bike path, watching robins and waving at rafters floating along the

Bow River. It felt like the best day of my life. Mom stayed upbeat. She had made up her mind, she said, to bloom where she was planted. The toy-waving women were good-hearted. Ella was a friend. The aides were simple people, but mostly kind. This was only part of the reality, I guessed, but who was I to invade Mom's fictions and convictions with my own observations of this warehouse? Surely she had her right to find her own way to adapt? When Judi returned, refreshed, I went back to the Coast. I was slightly less unsettled, and even slightly hopeful that things would be fine at last.

A month later I flew back to Calgary for Mom's first Care Conference at River Vista Manor. In this world of care, this meeting was a critical event. It determined what food Mom would get to eat, whether she would be washed in a tub or hosed down in a shower like some heifer at the Stampede, if she could leave River Vista Manor for visits home, and what drugs she would receive whenever she needed them, versus the ones that would be rationed, like her morphine. Judi and I had two requests. We accepted that since Mom needed a sling to be moved, there could be no soaking in a bathtub. Mom said she didn't want it anyway. The bathtub was in a linen closet with people going in and out and it was not her idea of pleasure. But the shower! It happened once a week. Those residents whose turn it was were trundled down the hall, naked and shivering under bathrobes, pushed along in commode chairs with their scrawny bottoms visible from behind, to wait their turn in line. The shower's temperature ranged between scalding and cold whenever the nearby toilet flushed. "Could Mom have warm towels to fend off the post-shower chill that set up her back spasms?" I asked. "And did the towels have to be so scratchy?" We learned that the pipes

165

at River Vista Manor were old and new plumbing was several budget years away. The lineups were inevitable as several residents "were done" on Mom's shower day. The linens were supplied by contract, so stiff towels were out of their control. "It is not a spa here," the Director sniffed.

"What about Sundaes on Saturday?" That was another stress. With limited staff on weekends, a volunteer pushed a cart containing ice cream from room to room. This was called an activity, and marked on the recreation white board for visitors to see. Judi asked why the volunteer pushed her cart past Mom without offering her some of the treat. "We have a policy," the Director intoned. "Residents with diabetes cannot have anything containing sugar." I tensed to argue but Judi squeezed my hand in that gesture that I knew meant stop. We must not get the reputation of being complainers. There were more important matters. What policy required Mom to be sent by ambulance to Emergency? It had happened twice already, for a nose bleed once and for results in some quick urine test that might have spelled infection. Neither were crises. Each time Lorne had called Judi to tell her to get to Emergency at one or the other hospital to be with Mom. "It is our policy," the Director said. "We feel it is better to be safe than sorry." Judi and I exchanged a glance. This wasn't about patient safety. It was River Vista Manor's concern for liability and its lack of trained staff to care for a nosebleed.

And what about the lockdowns? Judi asked. The periods where visitors were banned because of some spreading virus were by far the hardest for Mom to endure. She needed Judi. The Director shrugged. "We can't risk spreading disease."

I went back to the Coast, feeling demoralized. "Don't worry about me," Mom said as I tearfully hugged her good-bye.

"It's not as bad as you think. People are good here." If I was an expert at fibs, I knew I learned it from my mother.

Mom had strategies to make her way at River Vista Manor. The main one was to be compliant in every way, catching more flies with honey was how she put it. As a nurse herself, she knew how abuse could be underhanded but very real. Residents called feisty might have to wait just a little longer for their call bell to be answered. Their diapers might be changed a little less often. They might be spoken to sharply, or mocked with demeaning language: "Did you do another poo-poo?" Mom endured. Judi gnashed her teeth, but they shared another strategy. Both tried to see her situation through a spiritual lens in which everything happened for a reason. They said they "offered it up," that Catholic magic of putting suffering to work in a cause.

I wished I could move to Calgary. If only I could be with Mom at her meals, just her meals, I could make a difference. Being her guest, we would be able sit at the special table in the corner reserved for residents entertaining visitors. That would save her from the toy-waving women. I would offer conversation instead of silence. I could get her back to her bed when we were done and before the pain of sitting set in. She sometimes waited an hour for her turn to have the porter push her. I couldn't move to Calgary, so I begged anyone who said they loved Mom and lived in town to step up. Could they show their professed dedication to Mom at River Vista Manor at 5:00pm? I harangued, and everyone I asked demurred. I was being unreasonable. Didn't I realize that was the worst traffic time in Calgary? Of course an hour was too short for a proper visit. And dinner also had to be served at home. But underneath the variety of excuses was the one I knew was common to all of us. River Vista Manor was depressing.

Over months, Mom's care improved, if only slightly. She got a dollop of coffee ice cream when the Sundaes on Saturday cart came around. A priest learned that she was the mother of a Jesuit and began to bring communion once in a while. Warmed towels even appeared after her shower.

I shouldn't worry, she insisted, I should live my life on the Coast and visit when I could. Mom felt she was where she was meant to be. There was a reason for it all. God was in charge. God was in charge. We were excellent daughters and, once again, for good measure, God was in charge of it all.

13

Kidnapped!

"I haven't got much fight left in me."

The summer of 2008 slipped by. On the Coast, I tended my first organic vegetable garden. When people asked if I had goals, I shrugged and said that if I could grow just one carrot that was not deformed, I would deem my life worthwhile. I really didn't feel like talking too much about anything deeper than that. I practiced mindfulness and got pretty good at being in the moment. Back in Calgary, Judi shuttled back and forth all day between Mom and Dad, each dwindling without crisis on opposite ends of town. The four of us, main actors in the Parent Project, had found a rhythm of caring and being cared for, and felt the joy of surrender to life as it was.

But as the sumacs began to flame on the Coast and the salmon gathered in the creek below my house for their journeys home, I also felt the pull to Calgary. Judi was headed to China this time, her best business trip ever, she said with glee and anticipation. As always, I became Daughter on Deck while she was gone. Mom said in her wobbly voice on the phone that she was looking forward to my visit.

I also looked forward to a road trip with my husband. The two days driving through the Rockies to Calgary would be a pleasant interlude and give us time to talk. He planned to drop me in Calgary, then go on to Montana, and fish his way home to the Coast in every trout pool he could find. I would fly home once Judi was back from Shanghai.

My cell phone rang as we came through the mountains and back into range, close to our stop-off point for the night. We were half way to Calgary. Judi's voice message crackled with static and tension. "She's dying. Get here as fast as you can." I was stunned. Mom wasn't doing well? Wasn't she finally settled in River Vista Manor? Wasn't she peaceful at last? Dying? It couldn't be! I texted right back, just as the signal was lost again. "I am on my way."

Ed's jaw clenched. His hands gripped the steering wheel. "I am really tired," he pleaded. "I can't keep driving." I rolled my eyes. My head knew that his was healthy behavior. Rest was important. So was beer and a steak dinner. Everyone harped on that stupid rule that I must put my own mask on first. "And besides, it is dangerous driving at night. Moose, you know." Ed knew he was in hot water with me now.

"Mom is dying, for God's sake," I tried to keep the shrillness out of my voice. "Don't you think I am tired, too?" Ed cringed. "Drop me off at the bus station and stay the night if you must," I growled. We drove a few more miles in silence.

"All right," he conceded. "But you will have to drive."

I softened right away. "Of course, and we'll also stop for a steak in Lake Louise." We sailed past our planned stopover and on to the last big mountain pass, while Ed snored in the passenger seat. I drove with the windows rolled down to keep me alert enough to see the moose in time. My child inside was sobbing. Would Mom wait for me to get there to say good-bye? I thought about the tunnel filled with light, drawing her along.

"Please wait, Mom. Please Wait." I breathed this mantra, my eyes glued to the road. At 4 a.m. I left the mountains behind and soon looked at the mat of twinkling diamonds that were the lights of Calgary.

"Please, God, let me make it on time." Was that the child again, imploring? Was that a prayer? I laughed out loud. Magic words. That's all they were. Conjuring the right outcome. The outcome that suited me. Still, I felt a tiny balm of peacefulness. Perhaps it was the power of prayer.

"Faith is a gift," Mom told me once, when one of our conversations turned to what we believed. "I'm sorry you don't have it. Life is simpler for those of us who do." Only my brother John and Judi still held on to the Catholic certainties of our childhood. John grew up to be a priest. Judi grew up to be a thoroughly devoted divorcee. I had a spiritual side, of course. It was just not rule-bound like the Catholic faith seemed to be. I prayed again that I would have more time with Mom to talk about all this.

Ed jerked awake as I pulled into the eerily empty hospital parking lot. He said he would come with me to just say hi, then go with Jamie for more sleep. I knew he would do anything to avoid the stew of emotion we would find in that hospital room, and I was happy not to have him with me. I only wanted to be with Mom and Judi. The child inside was whining again. My adult self admonished, "You have no right of possession over Mom's death."

The elevator door opened on the unit. There was Judi. She was in her all-business mode. I hugged her and she pushed me away. She led us down the dimly-lit night-shift hall. Mom lay in the middle of an empty room that might have held two or three patients, her bed like the catafalque in Mao

Tse-tung's mausoleum. The hissing of oxygen and the beep of monitors was nerve-jangling Muzak. Chris lumbered over to me. He smiled but his eyes were dull. "Good to see you, Sis." We hugged and he looked at his watch. "Got to get some shuteye. Tomorrow is a work day." Ed bee-lined to Jamie to man-slap his son. Jamie held a thick textbook. Always multitasking, I noticed. He said he was cramming for an exam. This deathwatch came at a bad time, he admitted. He needed sleep. Within minutes of my arrival, I had my wish. We were alone.

Judi explained the immediate problem. Mom's kidneys were packing up. That meant she was bloated with fluid her cells needed but couldn't use. The fluid also pressed on her lungs so she gasped for air. She was in danger of a killer stroke or massive heart attack. A foggy plastic mask covered her mouth and nose. I leaned in to kiss her forehead and saw her lips all cracked with the blasting air.

"It's that damn UTI." Judi took the blame. She'd pressed for intravenous antibiotics the last time Mom had come down with a urinary tract infection. When Mom was sent home from Emergency like the last time and the time before, with a few Tylenol and a "See your family doc" kiss off, she had pushed for the powerful meds even though the doctor had warned that they might be too hard on a system so frail already. "I didn't want the revolving door to Emergency anymore," she said, and Mom agreed. "So we took the chance. The doses had to be infused once a day." Judi explained how, of course, River Vista Manor couldn't do anything as complex as delivering an antibiotic intravenously. "For ten days I lugged her every day back to the hospital. It was awful..." my twin paused and her eyes filled with tears, "just awful."

I waited and stroked Mom's arm till Judi could talk again. She explained how Mom stopped eating and drinking and kept saying she just felt lousy. But Judi admitted she didn't really listen. Mom always felt like hell, she said, and she felt this new low was the stress of the infusions. Once in Emergency, though, the resident found the thrush in the first minute. Mom's mouth was coated inside with white sores. Now Judi knew why she was not eating, and why she had become so weak so fast. Judi said she overheard the doctor fuming to the nurse at the computer kiosk. "You'd think a nursing home would find something so obvious," he had blustered. "Do they just assume old people go off their food? Do they just decide she must just be tired of living, for God's sake? Or sit on their hands and conclude she must be taking matters into her own hands?" Judi said she was surprised at how angry this doctor was, when he thought he was talking privately to a colleague, not using that different tone that went with talking to her, the distraught daughter. That balancing act between compassion and detachment, she thought, was that X factor that kept good doctors going. "She is so bloody de-conditioned!" he raged, slapping Mom's chart on the desk in frustration. Judi shrugged.

"I should have seen it. It was all my fault." As always, Judi rushed to take the blame, now for a condition that River Vista Manor should have caught right away. I needed to redirect her. She was beginning to cry again. That wouldn't help.

"Let's talk China. You are still going, I hope." I assured Judi that Mom was in a safe place and I would be with her every minute and Tom needed her now to be with him. I could see Judi's lips pressed closely together, and briefly noticed it was exactly the same grim glance of "don't want to hear this" that Mom so often had.

In this tension, the hospitalist entered. Her badge said Dr. Kim. She was an Asian woman in her thirties perhaps, with striking black eyes that held mine and shiny hair pulled back into a pony tail. I liked that. And I liked how her smile conveyed both empathy and sincerity. How was it that doctors could present themselves so differently just by their expression? Now Dr. Kim's eyes darted back and forth between us. She touched her lips in surprise and sucked in a breath of air, exhaling it in a giggle. "My God! I'm seeing double!" But then, she was all business, and her interest was not in us. She leaned right down to Mom, face to face so Mom could see and hear. "That's a hell of a good doctor," I nudged Judi. She nodded in agreement. 'Bedside manner' was our shared key cue of competence.

"Can you hear me, Mrs. Perry?" Mom did not respond. "You are in the Foothills Hospital and it is September 15th. You came here by ambulance. Your daughters are with you. How do you feel?" Mom did not reply. Dr. Kim looked at Judi and me again. "It's uncanny, you are so alike."

"What's happening, doctor?" I pressed. "Will she pull through? Is there a care plan?" I didn't want the twin chat now. "I've just got here from the Coast. Can you fill me in?"

"Your mother's body is shutting down," Dr. Kim explained. "Gosh! It's weird talking to you, it's like I'm talking to one person. Even your voice is the same."

"Shutting down?" That sounded so final. "What can you do for her?" My inner child was trying to take charge. But my inner adult was fighting back, filling the space inside my head with another question. Even so, I didn't ask it: "Should Dr. Kim do anything for Mom? Was this the time to just let her go?" Just thinking this flooded me with shame. My child repeated, "Can you cure her?"

Dr. Kim explained about reverse osmosis at a cellular level. Mom was dying of thirst but drowning at the same time. Good kidneys would sort that out, but Mom's kidneys were not up to the job. That was because they were full of infection, she went on to explain.

"What will you do?" I asked again.

"We can try to kick-start her kidneys with lots of protein. She hasn't been getting it for a long time. I recommend a feeding tube."

Mom had been feigning sleep. I saw her straining to hear. "Speak louder," I said, "she wants to be in on this." I wondered about this burst of energy. It was that thing they called life force, I guessed. Mom was hanging on, fighting back. Dr. Kim smiled to see it, too. "Mom sometimes pretends to be asleep when she just wants to be left alone," I explained. "She's not sleeping now."

"Feeding tube?" Mom rasped. I filled in her thought and asked Dr. Kim to explain what was involved.

"You will gag when we insert the tube. It will never feel comfortable. But as I see it, that is how we will get the nutrition into you fast. You aren't taking food or water. But without protein, you'll die."

"No tube," she whispered. I clarified that Mom would try to eat and drink, thrush or not, rather than endure the tube.

"What a fighter!" Judi marvelled.

"Yup, that's our mother. She's always been a fighter. Be tough. Suck it up! Don't give up! Stay strong!" I kissed Mom's forehead.

"I haven't got much fight left in me." Mom's voice felt like cotton now, muffled. "But I will eat if I must."

Dr. Kim was at it again, looking back and forth between Judi and me. "Who's in charge?"

"I am." We said it in one voice. Then we said, again on the same invisible cue and pointing at Mom, "She is." I gripped Judi's eyes with mine. "You are going to China." Judi took a long look at Mom, her lips working up to tears again. She made the decision I knew was such a hard one for her. "I'm leaving for Shanghai this morning, Mom, but I will be back in ten days. Will you wait for me?" I said I would text her condition every hour until things started to improve. It was our longtime routine when one of us was on the road. Our goodbye was a clutch. "It will be OK. Be strong," I said. She kissed me and kissed Mom. Then, without looking back, she was gone.

Mom and I were alone now, and I looked at the jug of green fluid the nurse had brought. "Seems you have to get this whole thing down by noon." Mom pulled the mask off her face. "Well let's get started." She leaned forward to suck a few ounces from a paper cup through a straw. We went on this way every few minutes and by noon the jug was empty. Dr. Kim was pleased. "Time for the next step," she said. It was a diuretic that would clear the fluid but its risk was putting too much pressure on Mom's heart. Did Mom agree to take the risk?

"Of course," Mom said. "You are the boss. Let's get on with it." An intravenous line was finally established into the back of Mom's gnarled hand, the nurse cursing under her breath that all the veins were collapsed. It dripped the drug that might save her or kill her. It saved her. Quarts of fluid began to trickle though her catheter into a bucket. When it was done, a faint new color began to glow in Mom's cheeks. I texted Judi. "She is better."

Over the next 24 hours, Mom moved from the green juice to a protein-laced milkshake. She chose strawberry. The day after, she actually smacked her lips as I spooned a soft boiled egg into her mouth. Mom said it was the most delicious breakfast she had ever eaten. Broths and scrambled eggs, pasta and even coffee ice cream were added over the next few days. Mom was a baby bird, opening her mouth to receive my offerings. It felt exquisitely intimate. She was sitting up now, watching CNN and eating. We both knew, though, that the infection was still raging. Was it time to call it quits, she wondered aloud. I shivered. I told her not to think like that, she was just tired. This was a setback, not the end. But as I admonished her not to give up, I wondered, what right did I have to tell her how to think?

The cultures grown from her urine came back. The infection was worse than ever. It was a bacterium that was drug-resistant. The UTI would never be cured and it would keep flaring up for no reason for the rest of her life. Dr. Kim was happy to see Mom looking better but she had bad news. "The infections team thinks we should not even try to beat this. The only antibiotic is a long shot and anyway, it is hard on any system. It could be deadly in yours. I'm sorry."

I asked what would happen, doing nothing. She admitted the prognosis was poor. She might have new back pain from the kidneys, over and above the pain she already had from the spinal stenosis. She would have much more fatigue, maybe hallucinations. She would need an indwelling catheter. "But we can try to treat the symptoms," Dr. Kim finished. Again she said, "So sorry."

A few days later, Dr. Kim came to say good-bye. She was taking time off and didn't expect to see us again. Her replacement was another young hospitalist whose name I never knew. He wanted to discuss Mom's Advance Care Directive. Was it time to shift from efforts to cure something that was incurable, or place the efforts on keeping Mom comfortable? He called it active care versus comfort care, and said there was a world of difference between the two. Comfort care was the more acceptable phrasing for palliative care, which bothered some people, he admitted. It was care offered at the end of life, when there was no expectation of a cure. "We need to consider where your mother is headed." I shuddered and my heart thudded with foreboding. "This cannot be fixed," he said again, to be sure I understood.

"I'll call the family," I replied. "This is a big one." The next morning, we all gathered around Mom's bed. The new doctor confirmed that Mom was doing well for now, but reminded her that the infection was powerful and permanent in her body and she would not be treated for it. She was just too frail even if there was an antibiotic that was a sure thing to kill this bug without killing her, too. Sadly, there was no such drug. In addition, she also had uncontrolled diabetes, hypertension, respiratory problems, and that unremitting pain leading to ever higher doses of opioids. Those stole her ability to think straight and bunged up her system in all sorts of uncomfortable ways. "It is quite a collection of chronic problems that you have, Mrs. Perry, and all we can offer for any of it is symptom relief. I'm afraid there is no cure for your kind of old age."

"Get to the point." Feisty Mom was in charge.

"You go, girl!" I thought. I loved this sparky part of Mom's personality. I hadn't seen it in a long time.

Jamie stepped in. "What do you recommend, Doctor?" He was the closest we had to a medical man in the family, a physiotherapist steeped in the hospital scene. "Mrs. Perry, do you understand that you are at the end of your life now?" Mom nodded yes. "There is no terminal point, of course, no one knows what your personal trajectory will be. But you are definitely dwindling, and faster than in the past." Mom nodded yes again. She knew the score.

"Doctor, before I run right out of gas, can we get to what is next?" She whispered her philosophy. She had had a tough life but had enjoyed it. She was proud of us. We seven children were her finest accomplishment. She knew she was loved. She loved us, too. Now Mom paused. Was she done speaking? No, there was more. Loving us, and being loved by us, was her purpose now. She wanted to stay alive to enjoy that part. But she was also tired, and knew she was a burden in our lives. "Everything comes to an end," she said. We were all silent for a time, taking this in. Mom went on. She added that she knew about hospitals. Her bed was needed for someone else who had a better chance than she did of making it and going on with life. "How can I say all that in that paper you are holding?"

We got down to business to change her Advanced Care Directive. At present it told Goliath to make all efforts to cure her, short of electric paddles to start her heart or a ventilator forced into her lungs to do the breathing. The change to Comfort Care would give a different order to the medical system. She wouldn't be shunted to the side, of course, and left to die, but efforts would shift to managing her pain and uncomfortable symptoms, and nothing more. There would be no more finger pricks and blood pressure cuffs, ambulances in the middle of the night, admissions to hospital, no more crises of the kind she had endured so often and barely survived this time. I read carefully through the document, twice. There was no doubt. This Advance Directive meant care to comfort her at the end of her life but nothing to prolong it.

Mom closed her eyes. Was she asleep? "It is important, however you decide, to direct all the energy you have left to what you value most. Your time might be very short."

"It's what I said," Mom repeated, her eyes still closed. "To love and be loved. That is all I want." The machines crackled in her silence now. Was she finished? Was that a smile? "And I never want to see this place again!" The tension broke.

A half hour later, Mom's chart was changed. She'd initialed the new box on her Advance Care Directive with Chris helping to guide her hand. Now that she was officially palliative, she gave us our marching orders. She wanted more priests around her than doctors. She wanted all the coffee ice cream she could eat with no more fussing about diabetes. She wanted us all to visit often. But she wanted lots of time alone. She had things to think about. She wanted to be with us. But even more, she also wanted to be with God.

"Contemplative nun at last, Mom?" I remembered her story, told to me eight years before, as we snuggled on the sofa in a snowstorm on the first day of the century. "Yes," Mom smiled. "Sort of like that."

A few days later, an ambulance took Mom back to River Vista Manor. We met Dr. Kim at the elevator coming back on the floor after her days off. "I did not want it to turn out this way," she said. I asked what she meant. "The medical system is failing you," she replied, wishing Mom and all of us well as the doors closed and she was gone. I was disturbed. Had Mom given up too soon? I imagined the debates there might be in the on-call lounges where doctors have time to face themselves and each other with the tricky parts of medicine. Cure at any cost? Or acceptance that Nature always wins in the end? What did it really mean, I wondered, "to do no harm?"

Mom resettled onto her same bed, but now the curtains stayed closed. Ella said she hadn't expected to see her again. Life went back to the same situation as it had been before. This was the problem. Nothing in her care plan changed except for stopping the medications that she had been taking in hopes of holding diabetes or hypertension at bay. The wheelchair still rolled her to the lonely dinner table, where she now picked at her food. Her pain medication schedule didn't quite take her to the next dose, yet each time she asked for more, she was told that only the doctor could prescribe it and she must wait. A country music band pounded incessantly outside her window. No rules were relaxed for us. "Of course you can't stay overnight," the Director huffed. "This is not a hotel."

Dr. Lindquist was as uneasy with Mom's changed Directive as Dr. Kim had been. Had Mom been manipulated by fear or family? He called Goliath's specialist for palliative care in nursing homes, a sunny-faced woman named Sharon. They asked me to leave them alone with Mom, and I watched from the door as they crouched on either side of her bed listening intently and murmuring. Afterwards, Sharon said, "Your mother is sharper than most people we expect to find in long-term care facilities," she began. She explained how Dr. Lindquist and Mom had parsed the subtleties of palliative care and debated euthanasia which Mom called mercy killing. Mom saw the dangers in comfort care as ethical and even moral problems. She wanted nothing done to bring her life to an end one minute before its God-directed moment of death. So she pressed that they explain the fine tuning between comfort care and euthanasia when it came to pain control. They agreed that morphine could be hair-trigger. Just a smidgen too little and there would still be pain and anxiety. A drop more and her breathing would become too shallow to keep her heart beating. "God is in charge," Mom had insisted.

"I get that," Sharon had countered.

"Her Advance Directive is appropriate," Dr. Lindquist also concluded. "She knows what it means, perhaps more deeply than I do." He added that River Vista Manor was not well set up to deliver palliative care. Doing it properly required much more staff, with a broader range of training, and perhaps even different values about living at the edge of life. The values were hard to shift, too. The focus of River Vista Manor was on length of days and safety, with quality of days taking second priority. It was not different from most long-term care places, though. Practice had a lot of catching up to do to respond to the needs of comfort care in most of the places Dr. Lindquist visited. It was a long-term challenge for Goliath to implement a new system and get it right. Mom did not have a long term to wait for that.

"How long might Mom live?" I asked Sharon when I saw her again. She didn't hesitate. "No one can say. She does not have a terminal diagnosis, but she is dwindling fast. Let me put it this way. In my experience, I would not be surprised at all if she died in three to six months."

"That seems right," Dr. Lindquist agreed. "Everything is wearing out and that UTI is one lousy break. It can turn into blood poisoning or lead to anything else in a flash."

I thanked Sharon at the door as I plugged in the code on the keypad to let her out. She said she felt blessed in the presence of Betty Perry. That was a new perspective for me. Not Mom the fighter any more, not the enduring Mom, but the accepter. No doubt about it, she was serene with her long time dying, I told Sharon. I said I also felt blessed. When she was gone, I texted Judi. "It's all good."

The next week was difficult, though. I called Sharon. Could she talk to the Director? She promised to have a quiet word with the boss of River Vista Manor, but held out little hope that things would change for Mom. "I'm so sorry."

Judi came straight from the airport to Mom's bedside. I stood back as Judi and Mom hugged and patted each other's faces, cooing in that dance of intimacy that belonged to the two of them alone and made me a little jealous. When we left, Judi raged just as I had been doing. "Damn that River Vista Manor!" I agreed it was not the best place for Mom at this point, but what could we do? We were silent as she drove.

"I can do a better job of washing her, flipping her, fluffing her pillows, bringing her juice and feeding her," I mused.

"Wouldn't it be great if she had more space for visitors now?" Judi added. We both knew it. An idea was forming in our heads at the same moment, as usual.

"Like her own room?" I said. We were coming to something. "She'd be able to sleep better at home, at least."

"And if it was up to me, she would have exactly the food she wanted exactly when she was hungry and it would be hot or cold and we could feed her in bed or in her recliner," Judi added. I felt her rising excitement. "She's in the wrong place for any of us," I agreed. Judi said she needed to focus on the turn. She hated driving. She hated left turns into traffic most of all. It was hard to concentrate with jet-lag off a flight from China, and these thoughts boiling. I should have taken the wheel, I castigated myself. She was in no shape for driving! Neither of us was thinking straight.

"Tell me again," Judi said once the coast was clear. "Did Sharon really think Mom wouldn't live more than a few months?"

"Yup, three to six is what she said." I hesitated. "You know, we could manage to look after her for that long." I paused again, glancing at Judi. "I'd stay in Calgary. Stay in her apartment. I'd be her primary family caregiver."

Judi smiled. We were babbling now, excited. "We'd get lots of help from Goliath. I know it has great Community Palliative Care with 24-hour on-call nurses." As we drove into the basement parking of the apartment, the 'why' and 'if' had shifted to the 'how'. How we would set up her room. How we would get all her friends and family to visit. How would we meet every one of her needs, head-on.

Are all significant decisions made in such a flash of insight? We were one mind in two, thinking together. How could this sync between us become a wrong choice?

Over Judi's first beer back in Canada, we talked about it some more. Of course the next steps would be difficult, but we were ready. If family did not agree, we would convince them. If Mom wavered that it was too much for us, we would assure her that doing it ourselves would be better than enduring more indignities from River Vista Manor. But we also knew that River Vista Manor would push back. They might never have experienced a resident leaving their care in any other way than feet first. If we needed to, we agreed, we would just kidnap Mom.

14

Home Hospice

"The patient has cancer and is expected to die…"

It wasn't exactly a kidnapping. Mom was never a prisoner in River Vista Manor. Still, everyone was appalled at first. My husband had a list of concerns. I wondered if they disguised what I suspected was his underlying problem: "I need you too. What about me?" I had no answer to give him. Jamie wondered where I would sleep, since he occupied the second bedroom. I assured him that of course he would stay where he was. I needed to sleep with Mom, in the corner of her room, so I could hear if she called for help. Chris said there was no way that they could visit Mom any more often. My niece Jennifer promised to help when she could, but her family life was busier than ever, she warned. Judi and I accepted that the burden of this decision was ours.

Dr. Lindquist agreed that home offered many advantages to Mom over an institution as a place to be now. He agreed to prepare her discharge papers from River Vista Manor with the magic words needed to get support from Goliath's Community Palliative Care team. That help would be crucial. The phrase that got Goliath's attention was simple. "The patient has cancer and is expected to die…" Dr. Nan was thrilled to take over as Mom's doctor again. Dr. Lindquist said good-bye. He worked only in the long-term-care facilities.

Any reservations I had melted in the warmth of Mom's delight. "My prayers are answered," she cooed, reaching out to squeeze both our hands. "My little nurses. I never thought I would see my home again. You are such good daughters." We knew the mother heist was the right next move in our Parent Project.

"You can't do that!" The Director sputtered. "Don't you understand? Your mother needs constant care! You have no training!" I lied as I assured her we had caregivers lined up the yin-yang that would handle everything. That hadn't happened yet, but I knew it would. Dr. Lindquist was on side with our plan, I assured her. "She leaves tomorrow."

"No way!" the Director retorted. "I need at least three days to get her records and her medications put together, the forms filled out, and the bills paid." She also said that if we took a breath while she did all that work, we might even reconsider this rash move.

"Tomorrow," I said again. "I have no time to talk about this, but thanks for your support. Excuse me, I have a lot to do."

Back in Mom's apartment, which we now called home hospice, Judi and I grunted and swore as we wiggled Mom's heavy electric fireplace from her living room to her bedroom. It was the centerpiece for our perfect room to die in. We took down the abstract paintings that might be scary now and hung family pictures instead. Out went her grey metal filing cabinet with papers that didn't matter and in came her favorite red velvet occasional chairs, the ones she had bought for visitors in better times. We recalled the shock of her caregiver, the

Blackfoot woman named Cheryl, who had gasped, "You paid what?" With the red chairs clustered around her bed, Mom was going to be happy in this room. We imagined a Norman Rockwell deathbed scene, with Mom at peace and surrounded by family. We didn't dare talk about how naive we might be. It was too late for second-guessing. Were we romanticizing the truth of what Mom's end might actually be all about? Neither of us wanted to go there, either. Instead, we swapped our memories of struggle and good times in our Parent Project. We planned how we would work as a twin team through this last phase. Who could we hire beyond what help Goliath offered to round out the support we would need? Would Donna still trim her nails? Would Maya still wash and cut her hair? Would Adele still come with her soothing massages?

Judi filled Mom's freezer with her favorite foods. There was clam chowder and scallops from La Pointe fish store, the tangy bits of herring from Safeway that Mom called rollmops, and vats of Häagen Dazs coffee ice cream.

Chris said he had not seen Mom so peppy in months. She watched him wrestle the La-Z-Boy and the TV out of her cell to go back to her living room. "This is my dream come true," she told him. "My prayers are answered."

He passed that comment on to me, saying, "…and we all hope it doesn't turn out to be a nightmare."

"Cold feet?" I whispered to Judi as we helped Mom into a wheelchair for the trip home.

"Yup, you?"

"Freezing. But I'm feeling the fear and we're doing it anyway, damn it." Mom squeezed Ella's hand as we paused for her to say good-bye. "I wish I had daughters like yours," her roommate said. Aides came to hug Mom, offering good luck wishes. I had a lump in my throat, and recognized it was not just the saying good-bye kind, but the nervousness, too. Were we doing the right thing? How would we actually manage the intimate parts of her care? I was ready to change her position and fluff her pillows and feed her and be with her as companion, but was I ready to change her diaper? Would I keep my cool through her hallucinations? What about the pain spikes that left Mom clutching her blankets and biting her lip? And then there was the fear of how I would handle the time when she would start to be actively dying.

Though joyous, Mom's move back to her apartment and into the hospital bed we rented for her was exhausting. She went into the same Rip Van Winkle sleep that went with every move to a new place, and Judi and I tried not to be concerned. It would be her last move, and just as well – they were hard on everyone. I yearned to sleep too, but was hyper-alert, as if I had an infant snuffling in the bed, not a mother. Judi insisted that we switch places for four hours each day, to give me a break in the routine. I used every second to sleep, sprawled on Judi's guest bed.

"Mom," I tapped her on the shoulder, "Barak Obama has won the election. Come see." Home hospice was a month old. Mom was awake more hours now, and seemed comfortable most of the time. She preferred the quiet of her room, watching the fire at night or the flicker of the candles we always lit. But this night was special. Long before any of us had heard of the name Barack Obama, Mom had been following his progress to the audacious destination of the White House. I knew she would not want to miss this moment. Her inner circle was in the living room watching the television. Chris and Linda had come, Jamie set aside his studies for the night, and there were Judi and me hovering around it all. Chris and Jamie helped Mom into her wheelchair and then eased her into her recliner, each move painful, though her groans also sounded to me like grunts of glee. I tucked a heating pad behind her back and hip and Mom said it was just perfect to get at the sorest spot. Judi brought her half a shot glass of Shooting Sherry and we all toasted Barack. As the fireworks burst over Washington, Mom raised her glass again, saying in a rusty voice, "Yes, we can!" Then she whispered to me that she wished to try to use the bathroom since she was up, and that I could stand by but she wanted to give it a go on her own. She'd been bedridden long enough now to be comfortable wearing diapers, so this throwback to an earlier time left me wondering. Was it one small way she could fight back against the dwindles? I strained my ears for any sound of trouble. There was not. She emerged, leaning heavily on her walker, pale and breathless, and inch by painful inch made it back to her recliner, with all of us holding our breath. Mom collapsed back into her chair and closed her eyes in relief. Then she sighed, "Yes, I suppose we can," and we all laughed. The night was a top moment in the home hospice adventure. Judi said that moments of togetherness like this was the reason we took the whole thing on. Everyone agreed that this living room beat River Vista Manor by a mile. Still, we all somehow knew that this would be the last time Mom was in this room and in her favourite chair.

I loved the priorities of the hospice movement. They were ours, too. Yes, of course, we focused on physical comfort. But even more, we tuned in to the fullness of family presence and friends and the comfort we all could take in knowing that this was the best it could be. Goliath's community based palliative care nurses were tender to us and efficient in meeting Mom's needs for pain and symptom relief. They reassured Judi and me that we were good little nurses. We were good daughters, too. We were just what Mom needed. When they came by they checked for problems like red marks that would become pressure sores, or the catheter tugging in a painful way, or whether bowels were working right. They also asked Judi and me how we were doing. Sleeping enough? Eating enough? Walking around the block at least from time to time? And round the clock, we knew that someone from Goliath's team was on the end of a phone. Like a home birth, a home death had its own timetable.

How did I manage? Every day, Tanya came. Mom had hired her in her post-GARP phase, a nurse who spent more than the necessary time because she liked Mom. I liked Tanya, too. She became one of my few friends in Calgary and we'd been out to lunch once or twice. Now she came each day to give Mom a bed bath and share an hour of friendship and reassurance that we were all doing fine. When other helpers came in, I felt better about leaving Mom to get the shopping done down the street at Safeway or the laundry down into the apartment building's basement. I used that time to call people who wanted to come for a visit, and make the special arrangements for family who all found a few days to come from wherever they were in the world. It was upbeat work. So was tracking down old connections from all Mom's earlier days as mother of young kids, good neighbor, Girl Guide boss, volunteer, woman of faith, and Queen of the Corner Office. Then there was the email bulletin that I sent out every few days, urging all on the address list to reply with their news, too. Matt had set up a Facebook group he called,

"We love Betty Perry," and I uploaded pictures if they showed Mom comfortable and awake. I made sure to share the warm vignettes of home hospice in all these communications, to balance out the evident reality that these were fading times. Yes, Mom's back still gives trouble, I would say, but yes, Mom still smacks her lips at lobster. Mostly, though, I saw my role as being with Mom. Was that a life lesson she was teaching me, about sitting in silence without needing to be doing something all the time?

Judi took care of the spiritual side of home hospice. She was at Mom's side each day at 10am when the Mass came live from Toronto on television. The curtains were drawn against the morning sun and the TV angled just so for Mom to see from what corner of her blacked-out eye still had vision. Then they said the rosary. Most of the time, Judi prayed aloud and Mom thought the prayers, moving the beads along. The parish priest visited, and promised he would be ready to come day or night for that final anointing when the time came. A parish volunteer brought communion.

In the morning after prayers, I offered Mom a tablespoon or two of scrambled eggs laced with cheese to add taste and protein, and a bit of buttery toast for fat. At first I tried to play classical music, but she didn't find that soothing, as I did. Instead she wanted CNN droning in the background. She called it her white noise. I read to her for many hours every day. In the morning it was the Calgary Herald's editorials, and letters to the editor. We thought of them as soap operas and they gave us something new from the crazy outside world to talk about in this peace of her bedroom. In the afternoon, we worked through historical novels like *Pillars of the Earth* and its sequel, *World without End*, all about the building of the great cathedrals. We also read non-fiction like *Guns, Germs and Steel*. Mom listened with her eyes closed, the heating pad soothing her back and hips and pillows placed to support her. One went under the crook of her neck, a thin one under her knees, and others to hold her shoulders in the semi-prone position when she was awake. When her mouth fell open and her breathing became a gentle snore, I lowered the bed and crept out of the room. I used what time Mom's naps gave me to stay in touch with my husband, lonely but accepting back on the Coast. I wanted him to be sure he was also in my mind while I was being Daughter on Deck. Wife at a Distance still cared for him! I assured my husband that I admired his ability to let me do what I needed to do here in Calgary. Perhaps our relationship got stronger. I wasn't sure and didn't think about it much. I tried to meditate but that didn't work. My mind filled any emptiness I tried to give it with job jar thoughts. Everyone said things like, "Take time for yourself," and I said I did. That was a lie. I realized I had lost the skill of relaxing, and though Mom was training me with the silent sitting hours, I knew I wasn't getting the hang of doing less to "just be more." My life path had valued doing, not just being.

Fortunately Mom had no complicated medical management. A bubble package of her pills doled them out morning, noon and night. They included laxatives, anti-nausea and anti-anxiety pills, sleep aids and the baseline pain pills to quell the throbbing that never stopped. The big guns for pain, her opioids, were separate and I gave them to her when she still complained of the fire or the stabs or the hammers pounding her body, or when I saw her non-verbal signs: eyes squinted shut and pursed lips. I kept a medication log to learn the circumstance of each spike, and fend off the fear I had of being responsible for an overdose that might kill her. How much was that last dose? How long did it take to bring down the pain? How long did the relief last? I was obsessed by oxycodone, fentanyl, trazadone, hydromorphone and morphine.

Visitors! The best part of home hospice was its atmosphere. If Mom was up for a visit the red chairs soon filled. If she was sleeping, I entertained the guests in the living room, bringing in the coffee or the beer or the wine, depending on who or when. Maybe Mom would wake, or maybe not. Every invitation had that proviso. If Mom wasn't up for being social, she never had to feign delight. I was firm on that. Mom's comfort trumped the visitors' convenience. Sometimes visitors arrived and left without even saying hello to Mom, and some of them never came back. Most learned to phone just before they were getting into their cars to drive over, for one last check that it would be a good time. When a visit happened, I settled the guest into the red chair, played the barista or bartender, but then withdrew. In an hour I checked and if I saw Mom's telltale signs of fatigue, I wound up the visit so Mom never had to send anyone away.

"Your mother is so wise!"

"Your mother is so funny!"

"Your mother is the reason I am a Canadian."

"Your mother is the reason I had my career."

"Your mother is a saint."

Judi and I captured these comments in a visitors' book to keep track of who came and how the visit was for them. Mom asked, "What did they say?" Sometimes I read the visitors' book to her as if it were a soothing bedtime story. Sometimes it triggered memories and, if she was up for talking, stories from her past. She said this reconnection with her past was one of the nice parts about being home.

There were good days and days that were not so good, and some days just had to be endured. But we were comfortable in a holding pattern now. One day, Judi's seven-year-old grandson Jaden visited. In his high-pitched child's voice, he said what we were all thinking now. "I keep coming to say good-bye to you Great-grandma, but you haven't died yet." Mom quipped that she was sorry about that. "I'm still here," she would say, feeling her arms and face where the old scars were. "Yup." Then she would assure Jaden that she would try harder to not be here the next time he came to visit.

Most jobs were routine, but they were never easy. Food needed to appear in those little windows of Mom's hunger, whether that was day or night. She couldn't move to get comfortable, so I had to get inside her body in my imagination, feeling what might be sore, to reposition pillows and inch her torso up or down, this way or that. She used a little Buddhist brass bell to tinkle the message she needed me, because her voice was almost gone. One more blanket or one less, a drink of water, a scratch on some itchy part, or just company and reassurance I was still around. I detested perineal care and changing her diaper or swabbing what pressure sores popped up no matter how hard I tried. But I got used to that, too.

Judi was able to work in her home office for several hours a day, getting what she called the flack work done. All her time away from the computer was with Mom downstairs or Dad across town. When I went to visit with Dad, Judi came to visit with Mom. Everyone called us the twin tag team. Jamie brought life into his grandmother's bedroom. He was busy with his job as a physiotherapist and his organic chemistry studies that he hoped would help him get into medical school someday, and his new volunteer work. He was a grizzly bear tracker in Banff National Park, looking for tufts of hair on trees or tracks in the mud over the few square miles of forest that was his beat. Mom loved to hear his stories and had a special energy when her grandson took time out to sit in the red chair and be with her. He filled a void that I could not. His stories came from an outside world that she would not see again and I had stopped noticing, too, viewing everything through the eyes of the little nurse. I appreciated how his sparkle rubbed off on her. He advised his grandma how to spare her energy to enjoy what good moments there were. "Think of your energy as a handful of marbles," he told her. "Everything you do costs one or two. You need to ration them and save the marbles for what matters most to you now." Jamie said that this is what he told his physiotherapy patients, too. It was all about balance.

Jamie got a kick out of Mom's hallucinations. They were part of her UTI and were no more harmful than dreams, he figured. I knew that, on an intellectual level at least, and sometimes even shared the humour in them, too. We both liked Mom's conviction that a gentleman caller was scaling the seventeen floors outside her window and gaining entry when we weren't looking. He tickled her in ways she hadn't been tickled since she was a girl, she said. The fellow wanted to take her away with him, but she informed him she was busy. Jamie and I tried to soothe her through the frightening ones. Taliban with guns were storming down the hall. Ghosts were dancing around on the ceiling. When she began to cry for a lost child, and would not stop calling out, "Who took my baby away?" Judi and I went to Walmart. We found a doll with the weight and floppiness of an infant, and wrapped it in a receiving blanket. With the doll tucked into her elbow, Mom was calm at last. We wondered what real baby that doll baby stood for, and knew it was just one more of Mom's secrets only hinted to us in dreams. Once in the middle of the night I woke with a start to the sound of a thump. There was Mom, on the floor beside her bed, in a ready-for-action pose aiming a phantom rifle. When conscious, she couldn't even turn herself in bed any more. In this state of paranoia she moved like a Navy Seal. It was a narco with a big sombrero, she was sure. Jamie figured it was his shadow crossing the hall to the bathroom that scared her. We helped her back to bed, and I bought a nightlight the next day.

Sometimes Jamie and I clashed. I couldn't take out my frustrations on Mom, so Jamie was an easy target. He had tensions, too. As the weeks went on, he began to suggest that home hospice was a big mistake. It was an all-day and all-night job. Grandma needed better care than River Vista Manor, of course, but she was far from dying. Sooner or later she would have to return to some long-term-care situation. How long would home hospice drag on? The idea of putting Mom away again made me furious. There was more. I could not admit to him my envy of what I saw as his carefree life, and resented him now for occupying the comfortable bedroom while I tossed and turned each night on an air mattress by Mom's window, always on edge. Most of all, I couldn't admit to being worn out, emotionally as well as physically. Late one evening, sleepwalking perhaps, I goofed. With Mom's catheter bag full of her cloudy urine full of floaters that the nurse said was pus, I staggered to the kitchen instead of the bathroom. I drained the whole bag into the sink, over a stack of dirty dishes. The acrid smell of urine filled the kitchen and startled me awake. As I saw my mistake, Jamie came into the apartment dressed in his running gear.

"What in hell are you doing, Mom?"

Now I was alert, as shocked and disgusted as Jamie was. No one could have been more shamed by this gaffe than me.

"That is so revolting!"

He was right, of course. I would have to throw out all those dishes, scrub the floor of the drips, spritz the air. But what I heard in that instant was, "You are so revolting." Me? Revolting? Of course I was. Jamie was right. I was completely disgusting.

I crumbled to the floor, gasping with the pent up sobs that only found their outlet in this moment. Jamie stood there, hands on his hips, saying nothing for a minute. He was shocked, as I was, and possibly considering what to do. I suppose he might have considered hugging me tenderly at that moment, telling me what a good mother and daughter I was. I needed to hear that. He could have acknowledged how hard this caregiving was for me. He must have seen that, too. Could he have promised to do more to help me? Jamie didn't do any of that. Instead he turned around, saying, "I'm going to have a shower. Get back to bed." I must have choked my tears back just enough to apologize to his retreating back. I don't remember. I don't remember cleaning up. That was my second-darkest hour.

My darkest hour also had to do with misplaced piss. It began when Goliath's palliative care nurse checked what was causing Mom's stinging pain, and found the tubing of her catheter dislodged. She shook her head and said that the Foley catheter must be replaced. She needed me to hold the light and splay Mom's legs apart. "It is going to hurt, Betty," she told Mom as she unwrapped the new device. "Starting now." Mom screamed as the swab of brown disinfectant began to sting her swollen tender flesh.

"Please make her stop, Janet! Owwwww...Owwwww... Owwwww! Why can't you make her stop?" Mom's considerable store of forbearance left her in that new pain. She was out of her mind with it, staring at me with pleading eyes as if this was a rack she was on, and I was her torturer. The light wavered in my hands but I gripped harder on her knees to hold them wide apart. "Why are you just standing there, do something! You are a bad daughter!" Was it ten hours or ten minutes or just ten seconds that this went on? The nurse said I was brave. She was as shaken as I was.

Home hospice eventually failed. I felt it was all my fault. The balance I needed to maintain between Mom's care and my self-preservation just didn't happen. I wore out. My health deteriorated. One day the nurse came by with a blood pressure cuff. She said it was my turn to be checked. She didn't like the numbers the first time. "Let's try it again." The second reading was worse. "How have you been feeling?" she asked.

"A little tired, I guess, worried sometimes, uh, anxious... but OK...I guess...yes, I'm OK for sure...I think...well, I'm really tired I guess. Why?"

"Well, these numbers say you are not OK." She explained that for some weeks there had been concern in her palliative care team about the long-term viability of our home hospice. Mom had started as one-person assist, even able to use a commode by the bed. Then she became two-person assist. Now she was fully bedridden, even needing help to change position. Her catheter was unstable and her skin was beginning to break down. Her bowels no longer delivered cement but acid liquid, so diaper changes were frequent now. Her pain was becoming impossible to manage.

"Your mother is still not actively dying, but we believe her condition is beyond what can be managed at home," the nurse revealed. I felt hot tears forming behind my eyes. She reassured me that we had done well. We had made a space for Mom to finish so many jobs of her life, connecting with all the family, being loved as never before in our care, and able to say things in the snippets of our conversations that had never been possible to say before. All that was success. Judi and I had to believe that, not take on guilt that home hospice had to end. The next step? The Community Palliative Team recommended that Mom be moved to a hospice well known for the quality of its end of life care. It took a week to arrange for that.

Judi and I were heavy-hearted as we waited, trying to identify and name all our emotions. In the end we agreed. We called our feeling 'dis-relief'. We were disappointed and relieved, both in the same sentiment.

Three months after Mom had come home to die, the paramedics rolled her down the hall one last time. The ambulance took her to a nonprofit hospice called Spirit House. Mom seemed to be asleep. Was that real, or was she shutting her eyes to shut out the world, and this new sorrow? She did that often now. It didn't matter. This transition was the hardest we two little nurses had yet had to endure. Of course she would feel the same.

"I'm so sorry, Mom," I murmured in her left ear as Judi gripped her right hand on the other side of the stretcher. "We will never leave you."

15

Long Time Dying

"I count my blessings."

The Coordinator of Spirit House waved from the front door as the ambulance arrived. She showed us to a private room at the end of a corridor that was decorated with live plants and soft chairs, night and day from River Vista Manor's dingy halls. "Welcome to Pussywillow," she said. "I hope your mother finds peace here." The paramedics shifted Mom's inert body onto a state-of-the-art hospital bed, with a mattress that hissed strangely. "It's pressure sensitive," the Coordinator explained, "so if your mother budges an inch, the support is redistributed. She will never suffer with another pressure sore." Pussywillow was as cozy and kitschy as its name. A handmade quilt covered the bed. Indirect lighting was controlled by dimmers. The art evoked pastoral serenity. On the window was a bird feeder, and sparrows fluttered around it, bringing their own natural energy. Two reclining chairs and a cot were ready for visitors. "Of course you can stay with your mother all the time. You are her most import-ant support system. Please consider yourself part of the care team." Judi and I were tearful as we thanked her. "I know," she said, patting Judi's hand. "It's hard."

"Make Today Matter" was the Spirit House motto. It was quilted into a large display in the lobby surrounded by butterflies, each engraved with the name of a donor. Bigger butterflies gave more money. It seemed everything in Spirit House was designed to make each day as comfortable as it could be, for everyone involved. Whereas River Vista Manor had a few plastic chairs for visiting, here there were nooks and crannies everywhere for people to gather in privacy. A fire crackled in the lounge, and just outside the French doors was a garden that even in December looked pretty. An old man who said his name was Benny was playing cabaret tunes on a grand piano. He'd been a swing band leader in his heyday and now just tickling the ivories gave him joy. He said he hoped to do it right up until the end. "Brain tumor." Benny was matter of fact. Then he smiled. "What can I play for you?"

How could two places, both with funding from Goliath, be so different? It made me feel angry. Was quality of life at the end of life really just a crapshoot? Some people wound up in a warehouse like River Vista Manor. Others at the same last stage came to a place like Spirit House. I was glad that Mom had hit the jackpot, but all places should be more like this than that.

Judi and I compared the little ways Spirit House was so much better than River Vista Manor had been. There were patient-centred touches like an ice-chip machine and a blanket warmer. For Mom they were luxuries, soothing her dry mouth and putting a quick end to her chills. The kitchen at Spirit House was tiny but it was stocked with simple snacks like cereal, yogurt, fruit cups and little pots of soup to heat and eat. Why was that so hard for River Vista Manor to arrange? The cookie jar? Well, that was different. Judi and I knew that needed a phalanx of volunteers to keep it filled. Spirit House had them. There were so many people drawn to help out in the hospice that there needed to be a coordinator of volunteers to make sure everyone stayed on track, and contributed their best gifts to where they were needed most. River Vista Manor had few volunteers, no visiting pet therapy dogs, and certainly no nuns expert in the art of the perfect prayer, like there were at Spirit House.

The Coordinator shared her philosophy. "Everyone has gifts to share," she said. "You might be the one receiving care, and the way you do that might be a gift. You might be on the giving end, with a different offering. But they are all gifts." I hadn't thought of caring as a gift exchange but the Coordinator proved to be right. The nurses and aides soon realized that when Mom was alert and able to communicate, they wanted to stop what they were doing, and listen. And, like me, Judi was surprised by the understanding that, though people gave Mom care, they received a kind of healing. Mom's words came slowly now, and she did not feel like talking often. But when she did, she spoke of virtues like acceptance, compassion, gratitude, and living in the moment.

"She's stretching my heart," one aide told me.

"She's given me a new perspective," another said.

"I asked her to pray for me and you know what? I received what I was praying for. Please thank her."

"Your mother is a saint."

Mom slept so much that I had time to share my own gifts beyond Mom's room. As a community organizer, I could see that the residents of Spirit House who were still mobile were actually a community of interest. Chatting by the fire with people like Benny, Mary, or Art, I learned that they were bored, just waiting, they said, for death to come and get them. We explored ideas of how to fix that, and they became enthused. A movie night with popcorn? A book club with someone coming from the library to read to them? Games night? Pizza night? Perfect! I helped them set up this self-support group. They called it The Smiles and Chuckles Club, and I could see it made a difference in their lives.

Judi was delighted by the chapel. The trims were in light-colored wood, which gave an atmosphere of elegance. Deep carpets also had aisles for beds to be rolled in. The stained glass cast hues of soft light over it all. A pulpit was beautifully carved with images for every faith. "There are services here every day, Mom," Judi told her, excited. "We can take you to Mass in your bed."

Mom smiled weakly. "That's nice, dear."

"Tomorrow. Let's go to Mass tomorrow."

Mom didn't get to Mass for the next two weeks, though. She slipped into the same Rip Van Winkle slumber as when she had gone to River Vista Manor, and when she went home. This time, it didn't last but was replaced by a disorientation far worse. Hallucinations left Mom panting in terror. She said ghosts hovered in the corners and they all had guns and swords. She was stranded in the middle of the ocean. Wild animals charged down the hall. Mom had no idea where she was, so Judi and I took turns spending the night on the cot beside her, and calming her each time she screamed. "Don't be concerned," a nurse soothed, "this is all normal. Changes like new routines, different people, unfamiliar noises, even the way light and shadow play on the walls at night are disorienting," she explained. One nurse had a different theory to account for Mom's state. She thought that she had an overactive subconscious. "There must be interior work she's still doing," she mused.

Judi found that out one night. It was her turn to stay with Mom. In the dim light of midnight, both sleepless, they were whispering about the places Mom had been in her life. Judi was stroking Mom's hand. As she reported it to me the next day, still shaken, Judi said she murmured something about how Mom's next move would be to heaven. Mom's head jerked up. She was fully alert and furiously manic in a flash, Judi said. "Her eyes were that dark flinty color, you know that look she gets when she is really mad about something…and her lips, the way they work…you know what I mean?" I said I did. Mom tried to get up, Judi went on. "She was leaving right then and there and told me to get off my duff and pack her suitcase. She would have no more of this malarkey. Who did I think I was?" Poor Judi, I thought, how upsetting that would be.

"It's good twin, bad twin all over again," I said ruefully. "But this sounds worse than the poisoned water. Then what?" Judi said she yanked the call cord and a nurse came running. She gave Mom a shot of something to calm her, and it worked. When Mom woke she said she'd dreamed she was being tossed on the trash heap. Judi said she blew her stack at that.

"I said heaven, for God's sake Mom, heaven! Not the garbage! You do want to go to heaven, don't you?" Judi said Mom withered with this scolding and of course that jolted Judi with guilt. Heaven was a serious business for both of them. And faith was their tightest connection.

"Yes, dear, of course I want to go to heaven." Judi tried to mimic Mom's timorous voice now, "Just that I'm not ready to go there yet." I laughed, and this got Judi started. We let the gift of mirth sweep us away for a while. Such times were rare and precious for us both. People who heard us do that said how weird it was, as the sound of our belly laughs were identical.

The priest came to offer the Sacrament of the Sick. "Isn't that the third time she's had the oil treatment?" I asked, "I thought there was a quota to Extreme Unction." Judi shot me with a look I knew was not loving.

"You have no damn respect about my religion, and it bugs me." I cringed, wishing I could take back those words.

"Besides, you are way out of date. No one calls the Sacrament of the Sick Extreme Unction any more."

"Sorry," I was abashed. But Judi wasn't done.

"So you don't know squat about what you are talking about!" she finished now and glared at me.

"I said I was sorry!"

"Well, you can just shut up. You piss me off."

I shriveled in shame, and backed off. Being on the outs with my twin twisted me inside. Through the years of the Parent Project we had worked through many disagreements but always avoided confrontation. We both ached now. We were silent for a time, feeling for a way out of this impasse neither of us wanted. Then Judi explained that Mom could get the sacrament as often as the ebb and flow of her illness required. There was no cap on God's blessings. I was so old-century to think otherwise. She said she was sorry that I didn't have her gift of Faith. I said I was sorry, too, and realized that was true. Mom had always been right. Faith made everything so much easier in crunch time. I knew our tiff was over.

It was Christmas. My husband and kids came from the Coast. We crowded into Mom's apartment with its furniture but nothing else of Mom's personality left. By the next month, the apartment would be gone. So the legacy art and knick-knacks had been distributed according to the little labels Judi and I had stuck on each item many months before. I admitted that being there shrouded me in sadness, even with my family around. Judi intervened.

"You need some fun. Take three days." She said she would take care of Mom and Dad and we could just go off someplace until the Spirit House turkey dinner scheduled for Christmas Eve. "Your family deserves to have some good time with you. They need you, too." Before I could think of all the reasons why not, Ed, Jamie and Fiona had started to plan to get us on the road. We chose Banff. It was not too far to get back quickly if Mom died. Yet it was not too close to tempt me back for anything less. We rented a car and gulped at the price of a hotel room that would contain us all in high season.

Those three days with my family were a kind of bliss I had not felt on any other vacation with them. I let myself forget everything but the moments we were in. We soaked in the stinky sulphur water of the Hot Springs. We took silly selfies dancing in the snow covering Two Jack Lake. We rode the Gondola to the top of Mount Norquay and shivered in the wind, telling jokes. There was a museum full of buffalo skulls. There were art galleries. We each ordered a huge steak at The Keg one night. I didn't think about Mom or Dad. I let myself be pampered in every way that my family's love could devise. When we came back, Fiona and I sprayed silver paint on a twisted branch we'd found in the Banff woods and wound a chain of cranberries around it. It was our Christmas gift to Mom and reminder of our togetherness.

On Christmas Eve, we pushed Mom's heavy bed down the hall from Pussywillow to the fireplace in the lounge. Volunteers were in charge of everything: the food, the carol singers, and even a quirky Santa Claus with his raspy "Ho-ho-ho's." It was tradition in my family to gorge on turkey with all its trimmings at Christmas and we did that now with gusto. Mom could only manage a nibble.

"I see she's pulling away from the world," a volunteer said. "It's beautiful." Jamie rolled his eyes. Was it the family being together that was beautiful? Was it our gluttony? Or was it dying? Fiona agreed with Jamie. Spirit House gave her the creeps. It made her feel like dying at Spirit House was like some kind of performance art.

I understood. To me, Spirit House was a cross between a convent and a spa. Bed baths were fragrant with lavender. Mom's body wasn't just slathered with lotion; it was gently massaged. The soft music in the halls drowned out sounds of clattering carts and cries of pain or fear from other rooms. Gear for patient care was camouflaged in eyelet lace covers. The rhythm of the care was tuned to Mom's waking, sleeping, pain and hunger. There were always people ready to pray with her or over her. Mom responded to Spirit House by not dying.

In late January, we served cupcakes and fruit juice for Mom's 86th birthday, after a special Mass where Mom received another Sacrament of the Sick. People we didn't know crowded in and that was just as we wanted it. Then Dr. Nan arrived. We had not seen her since home hospice. Once Mom was admitted to Spirit House, a palliative care specialist took charge. Now Dr. Nan was just Nan again, Mom's friend.

She gave Mom a bouquet of daisies, and leaned over to kiss her on the forehead. Then, in what seemed to be to be a stage whisper intended to be heard, she said, "You are a tough old bird, Betty, and you are not dying yet." Mom nodded weakly as she came out of her swoon and said, "I know."

Were those just words of hope from Dr. Nan? Or did she intend them to rat on Mom as a fraud in this place where people went to spend their last few days or weeks? "Yes, we count our blessings," I stammered, looking around and hoping that none of this exchange had been heard.

"I count my blessings," Mom echoed before she drifted off to sleep again.

I gasped to Judi, "Doesn't that woman know that if Mom's not dying, she can't be here?" I felt a sudden thud in my gut as I said this, and knew it was guilt. Perhaps Dr. Nan did think we twins were faking Mom's demise in a bid for better care. Whatever her reasons, I now hissed at Dr. Nan to keep those thoughts to herself please. The awkward moment passed. But I could not shake Nan's comment. She had reached a layer of uncertainty inside me about what was going on with Mom. Weeks had passed with Mom nowhere closer to actively dying than she had been the week before. Maybe it was true. Maybe we were pulling a fast one on Goliath. We knew the policy. Hospice care was offered in a six-month time frame. It was five-star end of life care in a three-star world, but it was rationed by an expiry date. Mom was dying, of course she was. She deserved the five-star care. So what if it was just not happening as fast as the policy set out? Weren't we supposed to rejoice that we had these unexpected weeks? Yet how could we rejoice to think of Mom being returned to the diffident care of River Vista Manor? We were deeply disturbed.

"It is not my time, girls," Mom might have said. We didn't give her the chance. After the garbage incident, we avoided all talk of dying with her. Perhaps that was so. More likely, all those medications she had been taking to keep her going might actually have been making her sick. Leaving the pandemonium of River Vista Manor behind certainly brought peace, and with that peace perhaps she was achieving longer survival. Whatever the reasons, Mom was occupying a bed and getting one of Goliath's scarcest resources, hospice care. Intended or not, Dr. Nan's remark had triggered feelings of foreboding in both Judi and me.

Our angst was right on. Mom was in the crosshairs of Goliath now, not meeting its six-month expiry date policy. In early March, the rumbling started. The Coordinator began to refer to Mom in a different way. Instead of saying, "She is not actively dying yet," she said, "she is medically stable now." She presented this as good news. "Aren't you fortunate that your mother has been given a new lease on life?" I had no answer I was prepared to give. In the deepest recess of my heart, I was thinking that Mom was taking too long to die. Of course admitting that would make me a bad daughter, though, so I could not share this thought with anyone, even Judi. Still, I wasn't surprised when Judi phoned me on the Coast in late March. Her voice had that familiar frantic tremble. "She's being decanted!"

"Decanted?" I let my fear be expressed in rage at the objectifying language Goliath so often chose to describe the people in its care. "Decanted? Mom is not cheap wine!"

"Chill, Janet." Judi said she needed me to stay calm because she was flipping out. We couldn't both do that. "Decanting is a lousy word. But it's not the point. I need you to do whatever it takes to keep her where she is. Work the phones. Find out how to get to the big boss. Threaten him! Advocate!" Our twin team went into action. In Calgary, Judi held Mom's hand more tightly, and ingratiated herself with the Spirit House staff. That, we reasoned, would make it easier for people with any wiggle room in the application of the policy to opt to help Mom stay. "You catch more flies with honey," I remembered Mom saying as her way to survive in River Vista Manor. Meanwhile, from the Coast, I turned up the heat in many directions to fight back. I sent out desperate emails and registered letters about Mom's 'case'. I challenged Goliath's pretense of patient-centred care. How could the system shuffle a suffering old lady around because her continuing to live was inconvenient? I quoted studies of relocation trauma in the elderly. I hinted that I would go public.

Someone in Goliath's superstructure said, "Hospice is not the right tool."

Someone else said, "I'm confused. Aren't you happy that your mother isn't dying?"

Yet another Goliath wonk said, "The nerve of you, thinking your mother can consume such a costly resource as hospice services. She has no right to that. She is bed-blocking!"

Finally, when someone at the end of the phone punched my deepest guilt button, I knew I was defeated. "What makes you think your mother is so special?"

I gave up. God would have to be in charge.

The ambulance came to transfer Mom in the predawn just before Easter. It was hours before Judi arrived for the day. I was studying plans for my vegetable patch when the phone rang. I knew before answering who it was. "Well?" My stomach clenched.

Her news was mixed. I must have touched some chord in the system somewhere. Mom was bumped from Pussy-willow. But she was decanted to a room in another hospice across town. It was a wing of a long-term care centre called Meadowland Villa. Goliath called it a chronic-care hospice. The existence of these dozen beds acknowledged that Mom was not alone in her predicament. Other patients were like her, too gradually dying, not meeting Goliath's policy guide-lines. Meadowland Villa had staff trained in palliative care. There were more nurses and aides than in long-term care. "Your mother is getting a higher level of contact hours," as someone explained, "because she needs them." On the other hand, there were none of Spirit House's patient-centered touches. The mattress was old technology, but we quickly said we would buy a pressure sensitive air mattress and leave it behind when Mom didn't need it any more. There were no ice-chip dispensers, no blanket warmers, no family kitch-ens and definitely no cookie jars. There was also no chapel. Though Meadowland Villa was miles ahead of River Vista Manor, it was miles short of Spirit House. And nothing came close to the care of home hospice. As always, Mom was sleep-ing, Judi said. I told Judi I was on my way. My next phone call was to the airline.

"It is what it is," Judi said as she greeted me at the airport the next day. Our hugs were clenches now, and lasted longer. I phoned Sharon, Goliath's specialist in palliative care whom I first met when she and Dr. Lindquist had grilled Mom in River Vista Manor about choosing comfort care. Sharon had started the hospice ball rolling for us. I told her about our failed attempt to keep Mom at home to die. We sipped our lattes leisurely, more as friends would. Sharon was pleased to know that Mom still lived, though she was surprised. She explained that death by dwindling was neither an exact way to pass, nor an easy one. There was no timetable, no firm termination date. She assured me that Judi and I were extending our mother's life by our care. "But at the end," she said, "you will be surprised. Death will come swiftly; from something you wouldn't think was serious. Her body will just say no more." Sharon gave examples from her week. A lady with a runny nose one day had pneumonia the next. Another old gal had a bedsore that infected and became blood poisoning. And just the day before, a man choked on a cracker going down the wrong way, and had a heart attack. I thanked her for her time. "Small things have big effects in this palliative world," Sharon said. "Keep on loving your mother and being her advocate. Those are your daughter jobs."

Spring became summer in 2009. Dying became just another way of living for Mom and the twin team. I reminded everyone in my email reports that now was the time to say what they wanted to say to Mom or to Dad, who was also becoming weak in Shady Pines. Summer became fall. Judi hired services that hospices didn't offer because the dying weren't supposed to last long enough to need them. Mom had nail trims and a haircut. But when Meadowland Villa's social worker suggested that physiotherapy might help Mom get some muscles moving again, "for her return to long-term care," our alarm bells started clanging.

But Dad was our main concern. People with dementia were not supposed to yearn for companionship. But Dad was painfully lonely. "His Martha" now visited only a few hours a week. She said she was out of gas for any more of Fred than that. Dad needed more people willing to talk to him in his now confused and rambling way. So Judi hired Brian. He was a retired engineer, like Dad. He drove a hay wagon at Heritage Park, all dressed up in a straw hat and overalls, but also did gigs for pay as a companion to lonely men in care centres who could afford his hourly rate. They hit it off. Dad loved to see pictures of Brian in his costume with the Clydesdales. Brian said Dad had wonderful stories which began to trickle out of somewhere long buried as they drank their coffee every Wednesday afternoon in the lounge of the dementia wing.

Dad had hated that lockup at first. That's what we all called it, not 'secure living' or 'memory care', which were Goliath's euphemisms. Dad said he liked the nurses, who were pretty and nice to him. We knew Dad was lost in a middle ground. He wasn't what Goliath called "cognitively intact" enough to manage upstairs, but had not become cognitively compromised enough to fit in with the downstairs crowd of dazed men and women. Everything Dad enjoyed about Shady Pines, like walking in the garden or listening to the cowboy music at happy hour, was not available to the residents in the lockup. It was painful to watch Dad suffer. Judi said, though, that the gap between Dad and the other denizens got smaller every month. His dementia was taking over.

At first Dad didn't need much extra care. He could get dressed and into his pajamas. He could find his way to his chair in the dining room. He could brush his teeth though not his dentures. He was willing to join activities like sticking something onto something else in crafts, or lifting his arms over his head and then reaching from his chair to the floor in the group exercise sessions. But then Judi noticed his monthly bill starting to go up. It meant Dad's needs for help in the activities of daily living were growing, and all were being charged a la carte, by the hour.

What worried us now was that Dad had become too weak to walk down the long hall from his room to anywhere else. A blood cancer, long since diagnosed but latent, was on the march. His specialist said it would not be treated aggressively because Mr. Perry was just too frail. Dad also wanted no part of more blood transfusions or chemotherapy. Since he was not able to sign the change to his Advance Care Directive, Judi did it as his agent for personal care. When she told him, he just said, "Yup."

I spent most of that second summer and into the fall going back and forth between the Coast and Calgary. At home I worked on my carrots, the one small area where my efforts showed direct results. I called it garden therapy. Judi and I talked every day. My last action before turning out the light was an email to her. The first thing I did in the morning was read her reply. When Judi travelled, I took over in Calgary. In her shoes, I learned how respected she was as a dutiful daughter, beyond what most staff expected to see from any family member. Staff liked her. She knew the names of their children and what their husbands did and where they were planning to go for vacation. I had no doubt. Relationship was Judi's special talent in the Parent Project. Mine was advocacy. Our twin team was functioning well and, just maybe, we were making a difference.

My days as Daughter on Deck followed Judi's pattern. I arrived at Meadowland Villa in time to tune into the TV mass. I read the paper and whatever historical mystery novels caught my interest. Mom was immobile, frozen, asleep. I was pretty sure she was not listening. Perhaps she drifted in and out. Perhaps what soothed her was just the sound of my voice. She rarely spoke. Her eyes squeezed shut sometimes or just gently closed at other times. Judi and I put her sunglasses on, and kept her curtains drawn because brightness hurt her eyes. When Chris and Linda visited, they opened the curtains and took off the glasses, saying that it made more sense for day to be different than night. Bright room or dim room, it didn't seem to matter much. I judged how Mom was by her expressions. Pursed lips meant discomfort. When her lips were working I assumed she wanted to say something and leaned close. I took her half-smile to mean she was out of pain and peaceful. Her breathing changed when she was sleeping deeply.

In my visits, whether she was appearing to sleep or not, I treated her as if she were awake. The nurses had no idea what this semi-coma was about. Locked in, someone hinted. I had several theories. Was she controlling her environment the only way she could? Was she in some state of enlightened consciousness, a kind of nirvana only really good meditators and old souls could hope to attain? My favorite theory was that Mom had her heart's desire, the life of a contemplative nun in that silent world no one could penetrate. Most of the time, she was praying for the world, I believed. I hoped that at least she was replaying the happy memories we had created together, like the time she wet her toes in the waves of the Pacific Ocean on our last adventure.

The food came pureed now. She sipped thickened water. I put a bit of glop on the tip of a baby spoon, and said, "Here comes a bite of chicken, Mom, open up!" As she moved the food around her mouth, I tickled her throat saying, "Swallow, Mom, time to swallow now." Every meal ended with a few

215

bites of coffee-flavored ice cream. All her life she was too fat, too diabetic, too busy, too poor to eat dessert. Now it could come first and often did. After lunch and pain pills, I set up her CD with Gregorian chant, the music that seemed most calming, kissed her forehead, and left for the afternoon. I dodged traffic across the city, knowing Dad would be waiting in his green leather recliner with the dents that fit his bottom. He didn't know which twin I was. It didn't matter. When his head slumped and he began to snore, dribbling spit down his chin, I slipped away. After dinner I went back to Meadowland Villa for the tuck-in visit. It was important to both Judi and me that the last words Mom heard as the lights went out at night were "I love you."

Mom had been in Meadowland Villa for six months when the rumbling started in earnest. The threatening words were the same as had proceeded her decanting from Spirit House. "Your mother is medically stable." Judi said no one denied that Mom was dying, though too slowly to fit the funding policy. Meadowland Villa had a budget crunch. A policy analyst deep in Goliath's bureaucracy had decided that chronic hospice beds were "not the right tool for the job." Long-term-care facilities should be able to deliver palliative care by now. So chronic hospice care at Meadowland Villa was an anachronism. Funding to sustain it was ending. To close the chronic-care hospice program down, though, one last bed had to be emptied. It was the bed that Mom occupied.

16

Advocate!

"God is in charge."

"**D**o not put me on a Procrustean bed, sir!" People said that Mom was one of a kind in her heyday occupying the Corner Office. Visitors who came now to visit the unresponsive form that had been a juicy and innovative Manager once, remembered her fondly as a fighter for what was right over what might be convenient to the upper echelons she called the mucky-mucks. They loved how she went head-to-head against those authorities and mocked them as snooty eggheads. Everyone laughed when they recalled her weapon of choice in those battles: words. Not just any words. Mom loved to use obscure quotes from literature to make her point. She found plenty of them in Shakespeare and Dickens. But her favorite source was Greek myth. She knew her adversaries would back right off, not necessarily because Mom was right, but because they didn't know what she was talking about and didn't want to look stupid. That was why the Procrustean bed image worked so well. In that myth, Procrustes was a shady hotelier who promised that any one of his beds would fit the customer perfectly, and did it by either stretching the hapless traveller who was too short, or cutting off the legs of the clients who were just too tall. A person forced to accept a policy that didn't fit was a victim of Procrustes. Like Mom was now. The policy might have been a good one – that was not the point. She was its unintended consequence. That was very much the focus of my advocacy now.

Actually I felt torn. My own career in a large bureaucracy, bigger than Goliath even, had been one of tough choices. Goliath had a mandate and a budget and had to make everything fit. There were winners and losers in every move Goliath made at a policy level. To make sure Mom would not be a loser, I would have to be a nimble David, scrappy but not too aggressive.

"For a start, Judi, don't sign anything," I advised her as we studied our strategy. "Stay out of sight of management. Don't get cornered by anyone who can tell you Mom is being bumped and then say afterward that you were informed." Judi started to giggle. Then I saw the funny side of this, too, and we both riffed on our images of Judi creeping from potted plant to potted plant in Meadowland Villa like some jungle commando. Laughing together about the ridiculousness of it all was one of our self-care strategies and we always took the time for that if something tickled our funny bones. Then we got back down to business. Mom must be kept in the dark. This cat and mouse game could go on and on, or come to nothing. Why set up worries that we might make unfounded if we got lucky?

My plan was three-pronged. If Mom must move, we could agree but insist it must be to Lacombe, the Catholic-run long-term care centre that she had singled out almost two years before. There she could revel in the convent atmosphere. I knew Mom would say her prayers were answered if she was going to Lacombe.

While pushing for Lacombe, I would send a letter of protest to the top dog in Goliath's system. He was not the Chief Executive Officer, though that was the power broker most often presented by the media as the face of the giant. It was the Chairman of the Board, who had policy oversight on everything and no one above him on the ladder but the Minister of Health. The Chairman wanted to be found, unlike the rest of Goliath officialdom, who hid behind assistants and secretaries who assiduously screened out calls from pushy people like me. He even had an email. It would be easy to reach him with my story of a dying old woman being decanted from her Procrustean bed. The third prong had risks. Would going public through the media actually backfire? Judi said she was nervous about that. What if public opinion turned out to be on the utilitarian side where what mattered was the greatest good for the greatest number and too bad for the losers? That would mean Betty Perry must move on. Just in case, we decided to hold back on bringing in the go-public journalists. We would use them as a credible threat, however.

I went after the Lacombe option and called Sister Ann. We'd been Girl Guides together. Her parents had been good friends of my parents when we were growing up. Now Sister Ann was on Lacombe's Board. That meant she had pull. I was grateful as she listened quietly to my story without interruption. I had to get it all out before I lost my nerve, or began to cry. "Mom feels like she is pulling a fast one just by staying alive," I finished. "Can Lacombe take her?"

Sister Ann agreed that I was right to have concerns for my mother's well-being, bounced around as she drifted in and out of Goliath's guidelines. She assured me that my job was to advocate for Mom. But she warned me that Goliath was mighty, and its mind seemed made up on this one. Was I prepared to lose? Sister Ann promised to do her best for a loyal and frail old Catholic, and try to crash the long line for a spot at Lacombe.

A week later, she phoned again. "Oh how I wish we could welcome your mother," she began. She explained how the Director already knew Mom well. Goliath had been by. She had a close look at Mom's file, and concluded Mom had too many needs, complicated ones, for her to fit in at Lacombe. "The Director thinks Goliath will have trouble finding any place to accept your mother, so stick to your guns." Sister Ann asked me to give Mom a special hug, and wished me luck. Scratch Lacombe.

Judi said her media acquaintances couldn't wait to tell Mom's story. A frail elder having the audacity to still be breathing after Goliath expected her to be long gone, and being bumped around like it was a game of musical chairs? Judi said Mom was a great hook for a media story about care gaps. It would hit the generation of boomers between the eyes, providing new reasons to fear for their own end-of-life vulnerability. But Judi's media contact agreed with the potential for backlash, making Goliath look good and us look like sore losers. Public opinion was not easy to control that way. Judi and I agreed to be circumspect with the media. But the Director of Meadowland Villa would not need to know that. Judi would ask how to bring a camera crew to Mom's bedside, and whether the cameras could take some B-roll around the institution. Fear of a firestorm was more effective than the firestorm itself.

My letter to the board chairman began with a quote from his boss, the Minister of Health. "We will be guided by common sense and listen to good ideas." In less than a page,

I told Mom's story and assured him that I understood what Goliath was up against. I quoted research about relocation trauma in frail elders. I reminded him that Mom was in hospice because Goliath had put her there. I shared what I knew about the fewer contact hours between patients and caregivers in long-term care, and referred to it in the words Goliath used, "degradation of care." I said that this was generally accepted by all the minions as a consequence of the move, but that I did not accept that. I ended with the plea. Don't disrupt this dying woman. Stop picking on my mother, or else!

I got an instant reply. It was carefully worded but clear. Mom would not be moved. At my computer on the Coast, I was yelping with delight as the phone rang. Judi had just heard the news. Advocating for Mom had paid off. In the Meadowland Villa staff, there was open rejoicing. For the next six months there was no more talk of moving and life for all of us went on as it had been for more than two years, bouncing between Mom and Dad, dwindling differently at opposite ends of Calgary.

We were in a routine now. Caregiving still filled up our lives, but there were angles we had not seen before. In fact, we felt we were the lucky daughters. Others, whose parents died without the long physical or mental degeneration, missed out. Sure, we had plenty of difficulties with slow dying, but we had special relationships with Mom and Dad and with each other that otherwise we would not have had.

"It's happening again." Judi was on the phone and I heard her telltale tones of frustration. Goliath had just chopped the funding for Mom's bed at Meadowland Villa. The Director had surprised her with this news. This long-term care centre was a business, not a charity, she reminded Judi, and residents had to pay their way. Meadowland Villa would not pay the extra costs of more staffing needed to tend to Mom. "Can we pay the difference?" I wondered. Judi said she'd tried that. There was something about Goliath's accounting that made it inconvenient for them. Paying more was not an option.

"They are calling her medically stable again," Judi muttered, "as if that's all the reason they need to boot her from her bed."

"I'm on it," I replied. We had a secret weapon to fight those weasel words. What did "medically stable" mean in the context of end of life, after all? We would fight using our own records.

"Before making any transfers," I told the Director in a long-distance call from the Coast, "I want to review all my mother's files since she entered Goliath's system." I knew that there might be many of those, scattered over River Vista Manor, Community Care, and Spirit House, as well as Meadowland Villa. They might be in warehouses. That would be fine. We wanted delay. I clarified that I knew Mom had a right to review her files. I said when they were ready, I would fly to Calgary to take care of that right away.

This was a filibuster. But I needed time to sort out our own records that went well beyond vital signs to observe vitality. Was that not a condition of medical stability, too? Why would medical measurements of vital signs trump quality of life ones at the end of life? For eighteen months, our twin team had tracked Mom's overall condition in daily detail. Keeping a journal gave us a feeling of control over something, and always helped us think more deeply about our response. Writing our joys and frustrations, as well as the daily observations, was a habit we both valued. Sometimes we would read the journal back to Mom like a story about herself. It was also feedback we used with staff that helped direct her care.

Using Goliath's pain-rating Likert scale, we gave Mom's eating, sleeping, eliminating, cognition, nausea, fatigue, mood and always pain a number between one and ten. One was the worst day imaginable. Ten was a great day, in our minds like the day she left GARP, full of hope for the future, and pain controlled without messing with her mind. It was all subjective, of course. But we supported our own qualitative data with a visitors' journal. It asked everyone who spent time with Mom to say something about the experience that day. "Your mother ate nothing," or "Your mother remembered me" or "We laughed..." helped validate our observations. It took me two weeks of work to analyze everything. By then I had converted all my fat files to one large line graph. It charted Mom's dwindling over 912 days in Goliath's world. Along the bottom of the graph were those days. The sheet unwound like a Dead Sea Scroll. On the vertical axis were the quality of life numbers one to ten. The line jagged up and down, and spikes and dips corresponded with what the diaries said. Overall I thought the line of dwindling looked like the trajectory of a kite without a wind. It was ever so slowly losing altitude. Her kite lifeline had not nose-dived yet, but it fluttered close to the ground. This graph did not tell a story of medical stability. When Goliath's files were collected I flew to Calgary and spent an afternoon in a windowless room in the basement of Meadowland Villa. Goliath had posted a watchdog to make sure I didn't remove anything from a file. She was impatient. "I only have an hour," she said.

"That's all I need," I replied. I didn't even need that long. The Goliath files were skinny, and became more so once Mom had become palliative. Occasional nurses' jottings were the only indication she was even seen by staff, and often they had to do with the inconveniences of taking care of Mom.

"Before going any further with plans to decant my mother, we need a Care Conference." Again, I shared Goliath's policy that this must happen before a significant change in the care plan. Arranging this took another month. Back on the Coast, I refined a strategy for the moment of truth, the meeting of minds I hoped.

"My mother must attend," I told the Director when I arrived. "We agree she is cognitively intact, though sleeping most of the time. Since this conference is about her, it must not happen without her."

"We can't do that!" the Director spluttered. "She's bed-ridden and on oxygen. Do you think we will roll her into the meeting room?"

"Yes," I replied. "I do. Just as the folks in Spirit House rolled her into Mass or down to the lounge for Christmas dinner." I said we would help. The Director accepted her defeat.

Two orderlies fiddled with the mattress so that it would not deflate when unplugged from the power source. They pushed Mom's bed to the top floor and down the hall to Meadowland Villa's conference room. Judi walked along beside, holding Mom's hand. I carried her catheter bag on the other, with the oxygen tank tucked in her covers. Mom seemed to sleep but I knew she was listening. My brother trailed behind, doing some last-minute business on his cell phone. I felt sorry for Chris. His job made mid-afternoon meetings like this one difficult to arrange. But we needed a man. Full family support facing Goliath was part of the strategy.

The room filled with a dozen participants who all had responsibility for some aspect of Mom's care, though only four had actually met her. I thought of the fable of the blind men and the elephant. Each man in the group touched the elephant in different ways to learn what it was like. One felt a tusk and argued that the elephant was like a sword. Another, finding a leg, argued that, no, this beast was like a tree. And so forth. Like the blind men, none of these participants in the meeting had the big picture of Betty Perry and, unless they collaborated to find a broader truth than their own perspective, the elephant would be seriously misunderstood. My job was to present that big picture, the one I knew no one would have in mind. Some of the participants greeted each other with small talk. Others did a double-take of all of us, and asked, "Are you twins?" Most just studied their Blackberries. Mom seemed to sleep. She was Exhibit A.

My tactics were simple. I would set the meeting firmly in the rights of this individual. Mom would not be a faceless file. I asked to speak first and introduce Mom. My goal, I said, was to present Mom as citizen with a past full of contribution to the community, not a case number. Judi passed around the portfolio of pictures we had prepared. They presented Mom as a wartime nurse, the manager who developed many of the health programs that Goliath was still using, and the mother of seven of us. I heard someone whistle at the picture of Mom with Mother Theresa. Other pictures showed her at each stage of her dwindling, with the shock of the Bullous pemphigoid blisters that ended her bid for living at home. She had had ten moves since that mistaken diagnosis. Judi passed out an abstract of my favorite study showing how relocation was traumatic for the elderly. The

Chairperson glanced at her watch. "Can you wind this up?"
I smiled.

"I'm done." The discussion began.

"Would this move be happening at all if there wasn't the policy change about chronic hospice?" one of the participants asked.

"Is this just an operational convenience?" echoed another. "Can't it just wait till she's passed on?" a third participant said. "We usually grandfather new policies when we can, don't we?"

I strained for names of these medical people, but there were no name tags and no introductions. Judi scribbled notes, catching these comments verbatim, I hoped.

"Hospice is not the right tool to use with this patient," a Goliath Administrator said. I jabbed Judi and she smiled. That old 'right tool' bromide. The Administrator was a tiny woman, but she seemed powerful in this group. Some cheeky grey-haired fellow in a rumpled denim shirt asked for clarification of the word 'tool' in respect to this situation, and I silently cheered. Most participants stayed silent. "This is an interesting case, no doubt about it," the Chairwoman summarized, "but we must decide how to handle this in the best overall interest of the system."

I raised my hand. "Can you explain Goliath's terminology, 'patient-centred'?" Judi leaped to her feet to pass out a page printed off Goliath's website confirming that this was its priority. No one looked at it. There was cynicism about the gulf between sound bites and realities day-to-day. And the website? No one was interested in Goliath's branding. Time was up. The Care Conference was over. Everyone rushed away, leaving us with the orderlies.

"You nailed it!" Chris chortled with delight. "Gotta go, though." He kissed Mom's forehead and squeezed her hand and dashed ahead of us while we rolled along in our unwieldy parade of inclusion. The nurse's aide was waiting to settle Mom back in her room. "Don't say I said this, but we all want to see your mother stay. She's wonderful to care for and," the aide added shyly, "we love to talk to her." I smiled and said thank you. But she had touched a nerve. "We love to talk to her?" Did Mom talk to nurse's aides but not to Judi and me? Why? The next time I was alone with Mom and found her eyes open, I asked her about this. "Why do you chat with the nurses and aides and even visitors who don't mean that much to you, but hardly ever peep when it is us with you? Are we doing something wrong? Are you mad at us?" I told Mom that we loved her, and that we too yearned to talk with her still.

"That's the point," Mom spoke with so many pauses that I concluded she had gone back into her fog. "I know you girls will still love me, even if I don't perform for you." I didn't understand. I was sadder than I had ever been when I returned to The Coast. I wanted to have all these hours holding Mom's hand be something more than mere presence. I hoped to smooth out all the ragged bits of my life with Mom since childhood, even heal that little girl still crying inside. Mom's muteness now felt like her manner when we were little kids hoping she would look up from her book and see us. Judi said I was overreacting. Perhaps I was grieving. I responded with a heavy heart. I just wanted a different relationship with Mom than I was getting. Am I asking for too much? "Yes," Judi said. "I think you are."

We hadn't won the day to keep Mom in Meadowland Villa. "She's moving as soon as they find a bed," Judi said. "We are back to square one."

"I'm going to ask for an Ethics Review," I told her. I had discovered the existence of a Working Group on Clinical Ethics, a province-wide initiative of Goliath. It mulled over such issues as Mom's long-time dying might raise. "At least trying to get onto the agenda of this Committee might buy us more time."

The Chairman of the Working Group was interested in Mom's story. Handling long-time dying and the degradation of care between hospice palliative care and what was found in long-term-care settings was getting to be an area of concern. Was Mom's predicament so unusual? There was a problem, the chairman said. Meadowland Villa must agree to participate.

At first the Director refused. Mrs. Perry's move was an operational matter, she insisted, not an ethical one. No staff at Meadowland Villa was willing to take this discussion on. What wheedling happened behind the scenes, I didn't know. But after a month the chairman called to say the meeting was on after all. There would be a time to gather the information, and finally pull the Working Group together from around the province. But soon. Mom slept on in her Procrustean bed.

I used the time on the Coast to study ethics in health care settings in the University of Google. I was humbled by the complexity of it all and saw the issues as far broader than my superficial desire to get the best for my mother.

I had many questions. Was there ageism in the society? Funds seemed far too small against the need for quality palliative care. Did Golaith understand that palliative care went beyond symptom control and addressed all parts of dying, the emotional and spiritual aspects as well the physical ones? Did the six-month rule about hospice care that we were fighting now actually mean that the all-round comfort care we wanted was being rationed? What made hospice feel to everyone inside and outside the system like a niche choice? Was it the branding of palliative care as care for dying rather than the best approach to all around support at the edge of life? Could people be trained to deliver sensitive palliative care? What was that training? Was it more a matter of instinct, compassion, or culture than a manual? What values needed to shift in health care so that 'fixing' would not be pursued beyond the point where cure was likely?

I had much bigger questions, though. If quality palliative care was so hard to find, or if people feared enduring suffering at the end of life, what alternatives would my generation of baby boomers begin to embrace? I knew the answer. There was an emerging option for those end days. The debate raged around words. Was it Assisted Suicide we were talking about or the gentler concept, Assisted Death? And what about Medical Assistance in Dying? Did that mean doctors and nurses and pharmacists would have to be involved no matter what their own beliefs? Would more and more boomers, seeing the unnecessary suffering of their parents, push for a new system that would support them in taking the manner and timing of death into their own hands when their turn came? We called it the Kool-Aid, the purple pill, the hemlock. It all meant the same thing, control.

It was a hot June day in 2010 when the Clinical Ethics Working Group met to consider the concerns raised by the story of Betty Perry. Judi and I shivered in the air-conditioning of the penthouse meeting room of Goliath's power tower. I looked out at the Rocky Mountains on the horizon, with my home several hundreds of miles beyond. I'd been on this dwindling road for more than a decade now, since that first day of the Millennium and my commitment to take on the Parent Project with Judi. One thing I knew for sure. If Mom had been left in her cubbyhole in River Vista Manor, she'd be long dead by now. Our twin team had been as efficient and dedicated as any family caregivers could be. But was our Parent Project really about death denial? Were we doing the right job in the Parent Project but for all the wrong reasons? Or were we doing the wrong job for all the right reasons? We had certainly been efficient. Had we been effective, though?

The meeting was called to order. Thirty professionals from all around the Province smiled as they waited for us to be introduced. I made a feeble joke.

"Have any of you ever met daughters so intent as we are on keeping our mother in a place where people go to die?"

No one laughed.

"It is ass backwards, isn't it?"

People studied their hands.

For the next hour, the group tossed their thoughts around. What was bed-blocking in the context Mom was in? Did she have no right to be in hospice because she did not die, even though no one said she would get better? Did Goliath's promises still have weight, if the operational situation changed? Was it assumed, or was it true, that long-term-care centres could not offer the same standard of palliative care as hospices did because they did not have the staff? Could that be fixed with funding? Was it fair to offer more care to some dying people like Mom if it could not be offered to everyone? Was equality the same thing as equity?

I was dizzy, tired, and getting that familiar feeling of blue. Judi and I were wasting all these people's time. We broke for coffee. Everyone milled around the spitting percolator waiting their turn. I said to no one in particular that Medically Assisted Death was getting traction in discussion with my acquaintances on the Coast, as the laws against it were being seriously considered by the Supreme Court of Canada. Did citizens of conservative Alberta show the same interest in this as citizens of my province did? Some people seemed to be listening as they sipped their coffee so I plunged on. If other boomers were like me, they might also be tempted to find ways to shortcut suffering and being a burden at the end of life. Terminal diagnosis from a disease, terminal reality from the inexorable dwindles. What was the difference? I wondered, if long-term care was seen by many as "a fate worse than death," then wouldn't they just pursue death if it was possible?

Judi jabbed me. "Not here!" she hissed. That was one of the few topics Judi and I could not easily discuss. We were firmly on opposite sides. She would have none of Physician Assisted Suicide as she called it. She felt it broke down societal values about cherishing life if it became too easy to put granny on an ice floe like she understood the Eskimos used to do, especially in times of famine. What was most important was that granny was the one to make the decision. She was afraid of the culture shift that would raise a new specter, "Duty to Die." Mom stood rock-firm saying God would decide the moment of her death. Dad had been well into dementia and could not express a view. I still wondered what he might have wanted if there was a choice for him when he could still think. He knew long before his end that the jig was up. He had a slowly fatal cancer, after all. I didn't want to upset Judi, so I just said, lamely to no one in particular, "That silver tsunami people talk about, I'm in it and I'm spooked. Especially now that I have seen what end-of-life care looks like up close and personal."

We reconvened, leaving the new questions hanging. "We will be preparing a report," the Chairman said at the end of another hour. He thanked Judi and me for our time.

It took another month for this report to arrive in draft. Judi and I combed through it and filled two pages with comments. The final version did not change. Meadowland Villa had to follow the direction of Goliath, its funder. The needs of the majority of patients at the end of their lives had to have priority over Mom's awkward but individual case. Promises were in the eye of the beholder. Besides, things changed. Still, every effort should be made to find an alternate location for Betty Perry with the same level of care that she needed and was getting in Meadowland Villa.

Judi and I were emotionally exhausted now. We accepted the inevitability of Mom's move. It would be OK, we felt. Mom slept most of the time. She said she was tired of the fight. "Whatever happens," she told us in her now faint voice, "just let it be. God is in charge."

In September 2010, orderlies rolled Mom into the elevator to another floor of Meadowland Villa. It was the Long-Term Care wing, but had three beds set aside for complex care and palliative cases, like Mom. One was available now. There were more staff than in the rest of the Long-Term Care, though fewer than there had been upstairs. Still, the new caregivers seemed to understand what Mom needed for her comfort and were ready to offer it. She still had a room of her own. We could visit any time and stay all night. This last decanting was the least traumatic of all.

As her second Christmas at Meadowland Villa loomed, there was another Care Conference. We didn't have to fight this time to have Mom participate from her bed. The new tone was collaborative. The pharmacist passed around Christmas cookies in the same tin that Mom had used to share her cookies two Christmases before. His wife had baked them for all of us in the room. There was the sound of munching and friendly chat around the conference table, as Mom's new doctor perched near her head, whispering something. He was checking her mental status, I assumed. I could see Mom was awake, talking slowly, with a wan but genuine smile.

"We were discussing Dickens," he reported to the group. "She has read all his novels and knows what characters she likes and why. I think she is more with it than I am." Everyone laughed. This was not the tension-filled kangaroo court of the last conference, but a genuine effort to find the best way to care for this woman in her changed circumstances.

Mom spoke for herself this time, with Judi listening to her whisper and relaying it louder to the group. Everyone leaned forward to hear. Mom said her care was tender and attentive and she was happy to be where she was. "God is in charge," she added.

Advocacy had succeeded.

17

Follow the Light

"I love you."

As Mom and Dad grew weaker, their tenderness towards Judi and me grew. They accepted our ministrations gratefully. We both felt a flow back and forth like a tide of loving and being loved. Caring and being cared for was now intertwined.

Dad's slide to the end began with a fall in December 2009. He got up in the middle of the night to tinkle and lost his balance. He crashed to the floor and sliced his forehead open on the unforgiving metal of his hospital bed. Chris said he was shocked when he phoned me on the Coast to tell me that Judi and Dad were in Emergency and she needed my advocacy help. "It looked like a crime scene in there, sis, with blood just everywhere." But Chris had several meetings that morning and couldn't talk. "Just phone her."

Just then, there was the ping on my computer to say that there was an email. It was Judi. She was sending this from the hospital. Dad was seen pretty quickly, she reported, much faster than ever before. That was the virtue of a scalp wound with plenty of blood. The doctor put sixteen stitches into Dad's bald head, but said he suspected a concussion, too, and maybe internal bleeding. Dad needed X-rays and proba-bly surgery to reduce the pressure. Judi refused. She showed the doctor Dad's Advance Care Directive saying he wanted nothing invasive any more.

"Well, we cure things here," the doctor said, "and so if surgery is not an option, I must discharge your father." That's when the trouble started. Her cellphone was down to two bars and she didn't have her charger. The problem was urgent. Judi had called the head nurse in Dad's memory care wing of Shady Pines to say that Dad was coming home. To her shock, she was forwarded to the Director of Shady Pines. There she learned that Fred Perry was not being allowed to return. She said his condition had been a problem of care for quite a few months. Now this new problem pushed his needs beyond what Assisted Living could handle. So now, Judi said, Dad was out on his ear: sore, cold, tired and now homeless. "You need to get to someone who can speak to the Director."

Bingo! He'd helped us before, when Mom was being turfed. He'd help again I was sure. And there was his cell-phone number! Such personal contact numbers were almost non-existent now in the cautious Web world. Things had changed that way in the decade since I had begun to engage with Goliath. He answered on the second ring, still before dawn in Calgary. I was impressed. I explained the crisis.

"It's not uncommon, sadly," Doctor Derick said, when he heard the story. "Assisted living gets to be inappropriate as its residents dwindle further, but it is often hard to uproot them." He asked where Dad was now. I heard him whistle when I said Dad was marooned in a discharge lounge with Judi and I was calling from a time zone away because she could not use her phone to reach him just a few blocks away from the hospital. "Tell your sister to hang tight, I'll see if I can talk to the Director of Shady Pines." It took two hours to hear again from him, while I paced on the Coast and Judi prayed while she held Dad's hand in the chilly discharge lounge near the winter drafts of the hospital exit. Just as Judi's cell phone went dead, I was able to tell her that yes, she could take Dad back to his familiar room, the one he called his wicki-up, and then she must meet with the Director to seek a more permanent solution. It was a start.

Judi was able to talk the Director into letting Dad stay, but it was a hard bargain. Shady Pines was a business and to keep Dad in this new situation, there had to be a lot more money changing hands for his care. Furthermore, family must agree to stay with him, at night especially, when staff levels were low. "Can you come right away?" Judi asked. "Dad needs you to be his night nurse."

I cancelled a Christmas party and phoned my sister Nancy in Vancouver. She didn't hesitate, either. We would meet at the airport and travel together to Calgary, Judi's badly needed reinforcements. Dad would have a formidable family team, in fact, three daughters, Chris and Linda, and Dad's grandchildren Jennifer and Jamie. Judi prepared a visiting schedule and Nancy took days while I took nights to begin with.

Dad had no memory of his fall. He said he had never been so tired and cold. He was thrilled to see everyone, though. It took some time to name us, but when we reminded him of who we are, he said "Ooooh," and remembered us after that. Nancy and I had our special ways to be with Dad, and knew our time would be difficult, but precious. If there was pressure building in his head, it would not be long before something even worse than his fall happened. A stroke perhaps. A heart attack. I hoped that whatever it would be, his end would be quick. Then I stopped myself. "Wasn't this negative thinking? Wildly premature?" Nancy went through Dad's tattered address book with him and culled the names of everyone who was dead. Would Dad like to send Christmas greetings to those who remained? He would. For two days they dredged what memory they could from his broken mind and wrote notes. "What would you like to say?" Nancy asked each time.

Each time, Dad had the same answer. "Say, 'I love you'." Then Dad signed all the cards with his wiggly 'X'. They mailed them in the box by Shady Pines' front door.

"You do it, Dad," Nancy said, and snapped a picture. Pushing him back to his room in his wheelchair, they sang the only fragment of a song that Dad still knew: "It's a Long Way to Tipperary." He whispered the one line he was sure of in his gravelly voice, "My heart's right there." Dad was dead before those Christmas greetings arrived. Her photograph of Dad leaning into the post box was the last one taken of him alive.

I took the night shift. In the evenings we looked at the digital frame with all the family pictures. I slowed it down to give me lots of time to point to everyone and remind Dad who they were. "Oooooh," he said each time a new picture came up. At bedtime, Dad was too restless to sleep. It was the coldest part of the year, and frost was thick on the inside corners of his windows, which creaked in the howling wind. I put his duvet on him because he shivered with cold, but he yanked it off, sweating, over and over all night. Dad wanted to be naked and he needed to tinkle. Up and down, up and down we went while he mumbled his confusion. Where was he? Where was his Martha? Why was I with him? Was I Judi or Janet? We spent several nights in this sad dance.

What held me back from climbing into the bed beside my father those cold nights? I could have cuddled him and protected him and kept him warm. I could have reassured him he was not alone, and that he was loved. What was my fear? In the deepest recess of my heart, where my child lived, I knew. If he brushed me away that child would be rejected and I was not willing to take that risk now that we were at the extreme edge of his life. I was such a coward! Dad needed me to be braver than that! Still, I held back. From the floor beside the bed I crooned, "Go to sleep, Dad. I love you, Dad. I am here, Dad. You are not alone, Dad."

After a week, I was exhausted and needed to deal with the work of Christmas on the Coast. I flew home, with Nancy. For three days Judi shuttled between Mom and Dad, sliding on the treacherous winter roads too cold for sanding now and taking her place on the floor beside Dad at night, just as I had been doing.

Mom was alert only once in Dad's actively dying time. Judi told her what had happened and that Dad would probably not recover. She was silent for so long that Judi told me she wondered if Mom hadn't heard, or didn't care.

"I'm sorry," was all Mom said.

Was she sorry that Judi was upset? Was she sorry that Dad was dying? Or did she regret her years of anger? Judi didn't know. She said she chose to believe that those two words were a statement of forgiveness. Time had run out for anything more than that. The reconciliation with Betty that Dad yearned for would not happen now.

"You need rest," the head nurse told Judi when she saw her, almost sleepwalking from Dad's room. She told Judi to take the night off. She promised to add more staff to keep watch over Fred. Judi was grateful for the night in her own bed. Besides, she had seen Martha pull into the parking lot. It was his time to be with his wife. He would not be alone.

Before the sun had risen the next day, Judi got the call. Martha had left after an hour. Dad had died in the night. Checking at 4 a.m. the nurse noted Dad was sleeping peacefully on his side with his hands tucked under his cheek, like a child, warm under his duvet. He was snoring lightly, the nurse said. All was well. At 6 a.m., when she checked again, Dad was cold. The Nurse said some people just didn't want anyone around when they passed. Dad must have taken his opportunity to start his journey from the edge of life in his own way, following the light.

Judi said the hardest part was watching his body be taken away later that morning. He had bought and paid for no frills, but that meant that Dad was moved like something no longer valuable headed for shredding. Two men in jeans zipped his body into a bag and rolled him on the squeaky gurney with loose wheels spinning to the loading dock and into a rusty cargo van. Now he lay in the warehouse on the outskirts of the city where the next step, cremation, would happen after we identified Dad's remains. "You and Nancy, get back as soon as you can," Judi said. "We must do this together."

The mortician at the warehouse was more presentable. She offered her condolences and ushered us into the back room. Soon a gurney was rolled out of a door that seemed to be cold storage. Chris pulled back the corner of the sheet. Dad's face was alabaster and his wrinkles were flattened now. It was definitely Dad, but Dad was definitely gone, along with the animating energy of his life. The pajama top he'd kept tearing off in his last week was now buttoned around his neck. Nancy snapped too many pictures, saying she was doing a project. Chris checked his watch and said his toes were getting numb in the cold. Were they saving money by turning off the heat, he wondered? Judi just stared, her hands clasped in a way I knew meant prayer. I lifted the sheet that covered Dad's legs, wondering if his whole body looked like marble. There was a tag, twist-tied to his toe. "Fred Perry," it said. And on his calf, scrawled in grease pen, was "Perry." That struck us all as funny. Chris thought the old man would have cracked up, too. We started by laughing, but soon were dabbing our eyes and hugging each other. Dad deserved sorrow.

The funeral went according to Dad's detailed plans. The teenage electric guitar player stomped out cowboy hymns. Ben the elegist used our stories to craft an upbeat speech. The sandwiches were all egg salad. Pastor Julie admitted she was never so happy to close a file, and would always have a soft spot for her most quirky congregant ever.

Judi kept Dad's shoebox of ashes in her closet until the next summer. Dad had set out one more job for us. We needed to spread his ashes in the swamp. John stayed with Mom in Calgary. This was not a Christian interment and he could not participate. Anyway, someone had to be with Mom. The rest of us met in a parking lot at the edge of a fen near the Vancouver airport. Dad had turned his interment into an offbeat family adventure. Nancy read out the directions we were to follow as if we were geocaching. Which bus stop? How many telephone poles along the path to the pond where he wanted to spend eternity? Which rocky outcrop would Matt stand on and what direction must he face to avoid the wind blowing Dad's cremains back into all our eyes? We were a parade of family and friends with Matt in the lead, wearing Dad's safari hat and carrying the box aloft. I kept watch for police. Spreading ashes was illegal, especially in a protected area for wildlife. We sang Dad's playlist of campfire songs but stopped when someone suggested "99 Bottles of Beer on the Wall." It wasn't seemly. I took a jar of Dad's grit before Matt hurled the rest into the calm water, sending the gaggle of Canada geese flying. When I got back to the Coast, I spread my jar of Dad's remains into a canyon near my house. It was my own place to be with Dad's spirit.

A year later, Mom died.

Her appetite disappeared in the last weeks. There was a family feud over whether to feed her or not. "Why do you keep doing that, Mom?" Judi's daughter Jennifer stormed. "Can't you see that this is her way to control her end?" Judi and I didn't see it that way. So someone stood with Mom at every meal, encouraging a spoonful or two of puree. Mom always seemed to respond to the cold feel of the coffee ice cream.

She slept now most of the time. I imagined her in a deep meditative state, or sifting through her memories or making sense of her life in dreams. Perhaps she was praying for the world. Everyone agreed on one thing. Mom was at peace. A steady trickle of morphine kept pain at bay. Some of the nurses thought that her deeply depressed cognition was because of that narcotic. Others didn't care. Judi read her Advance Care Directive to say that it was OK. But no intentional overdose! God was in charge, not a well-meaning physician.

Everything was in a holding pattern now. I wanted to get going on a long-held-off personal goal to speak Spanish. I needed to do this. My daughter was in love with a Mexican whose family spoke no English. Language immersion was an important family matter now. My mission. It seemed to be a good time to go after that. So my husband and I planned to spend three months in Mexico in an immersion program. I went to Calgary as Daughter on Deck before I left to be the backup for Judi on a business trip, and to say goodbye for a while. I quivered as I kissed Mom's forehead and shared my plan, promising to see her in the spring. She didn't open her eyes, but was it my imagination? I think she squeezed my hand. And was that half grimace fleeting across her face really a smile? I know she heard me, and knew it was me beside her. So I was sure it was not my imagination when she mouthed the words, "Be happy." What did "happy" mean, though? Certainly she did not mean the happy of a good meal or a day at the beach. Was it the learning and loving kind of happy that drove her through life? I knew. If Mom could wake and squeeze my hand and talk to me about what was important in life, I knew what she would say. I must learn Spanish.

"I will," I said. I was on my way.

Dad picked his time to die when he was alone. Did Mom also choose her time, waiting until I gave that sign I was ready to move on?

Along the interstates to Dallas where we were picking up our flight to Mexico, I kept my cellphone in my hand. Texts flew non-stop between Judi and me. In truck stops a long email told me Chris had brought Mom a soft ice cream cone for her 88th birthday and she licked it. She opened her eyes for a few minutes and told Judi she had many visitors in the room, her mother, her father, her brothers. Judi said that she agreed that everyone was gathering in heaven for the big welcome home. It put a big lump in her throat, she admitted. The doctor had told Judi that Mom was actively dying. Hydration might give her comfort. Was Judi OK with an intravenous? Judi asked if it would give Mom more time. "No," the doctor said, "but it will make her more comfortable." Judi said yes, of course. Comfort. Comfort. Comfort. It was all about comfort now. Sadly, Mom's body could not absorb this fluid. It made her agitated so she needed more morphine. Her vital signs were wavering. What was I doing flying to Mexico, I wondered, when Mom lay dying? What irony had me headed away from Judi in her hour of need? Ed pressed me to stick with the plan. He'd seen too many deathbed scenes with his mother-in-law to believe this was really the end. She would recover, he insisted. The texts went on.

"We are saying the rosary."

"I am playing Gregorian chant."

"I found the priest and he came."

"She's in a coma."

Then, I got a message with a row of exclamation marks. "Mom said she loves me!!!!"

"Of course she loves you Judi," I texted right back. So, "I love you" were Mom's last words.

I was unpacking in our tiny bedroom in Mexico, irritated already by barking dogs, creaking fans, and my husband practicing his hundred words of Spanish with the señora as if this tragedy were not unfolding for me. I wanted to be alone but I wished he would capture my mood and stay with me emotionally. I needed a hug, but he was not that sort of man. I felt isolated, weepy, scared. The cellphone jangled. It was Judi. She put the receiver to Mom's mouth. "Listen to this," she said. "What do you think?" Judi was the boiled frog. She was too close to the scene to hear what I couldn't miss from where I sat cross legged on my bed in Mexico. "Isn't that what they call a death rattle? I'm coming."

My husband grumbled. He reminded me of all the other times Mom was dying. Why was this time different? He needed me to stay with him. Just this once, could I choose him and help him pull off this challenge of Spanish immersion? "I'll be back," I assured him. My plane was on the runway when the last text before turning off my phone arrived. It said, "She's gone."

Judi was alone with Mom at Meadowland Villa the night she died. Chris and Linda had gone home for a nap. The nurse couldn't offer hope, but she brought tea. She said there would be several more hours before the end.

She was wrong.

In Houston I read Judi's description of Mom's last hours. "There were long gaps in those breaths you heard. I held her hand and it was getting cold. I fell asleep, with my head on her chest in an awkward position. I was trying to hug her. I woke with a jolt, and a stiff neck. Something felt different." I knew Judi needed to go through every bit of the story and I needed her to do that. "She wasn't breathing. I kissed her. I felt her lips fluttering, kissing me back. I'm not sure, but yes, I think she kissed me back."

"Of course she kissed you, Judi," I texted her. "She kissed me, too. She said good bye to both of us."

"Then Mom followed the light." Judi couldn't talk more. She just wanted to be quiet with Mom until the funeral directors took her away. She said the staff had said she could take all the time she needed. "We won't fill the bed again today," her message ended.

244

The airplane doors closed and I was alone with myself. I sorted through my feelings as I sat, my forehead to the window over the wing, looking at the passing clouds below. I recognized jealousy. It wasn't fair. Judi had been the first to see Mom when we were born, and now she was the last to see her at the end. Hard on the feeling of jealousy came guilt. I hadn't gone the distance. Finally, there was the heart-tight feeling I knew was the beginning of grief. By the time I was greeted by Judi's husband Tom in arrivals, my sadness had become relief. That, and a feeling that I recognized as peacefulness. It was over.

I found Judi and Chris cleaning out Mom's room at Meadowland Villa. Her crosses and pictures, Kleenex and creams went into a box. I fingered the soft little baby brush, that focal point for Judi's sorrow that I knew would always be her odd but cherished keepsake. She'd taken away Mom's bristly hair brush, saying it was hard on her scalp. Mom protested that she liked its scratch. "But I knew best," Judi said now, castigating herself as she fingered its flimsiness, and sighed. "What a bitch I was."

"Poor Mom, we were such bossy twins," I agreed.

Residents milled around, leaning on their walkers, saying they were sorry for our loss, but wondering what we were going to do with her stuff. They were vultures, Chris said, disgusted.

"Are you taking the TV?"

"I love those pretty nighties with the Velcro."

"Can I have that pillow?"

"I could sure use that extra chair."

"Do you need that blanket?"

"That plant is nice. Can I have it?"

In long-term care, life dragged for those not actively dying. Mom's last gesture was a free store and it spread a kind of joy. It was easy to leave Meadowland Villa and end our long relationship with Goliath.

As with Dad the year before, we were required to confirm that Elizabeth Therese Perry was under the sheet. She was. We left a packet of her make-up with the funeral director. We also left some clothes for her to wear for the private viewing. We'd picked them out months before, noting a coffee stain and having one of our can't-get-breath laughing fits just imagining Mom wincing in her coffin.

Daughter on Deck and Daughter at a Distance had no time to cry. As it had always been through the Parent Project, our siblings expected our leadership in making and implementing arrangements. We did Mom proud on that. The night before the funeral, her seven kids sat cross-legged on all the beds in the double room at the hotel and watched the Betty show. The DVD with all the pictures strung together in a life well lived had been ready for years, but the last addition was the death date. The bathtub was full of cans of beer on ice, that touch Judi insisted was a family tradition whether we actually drank it or not. The connected rooms reeked of pepperoni pizza. Grandchildren played video games in one room and great grandchildren played tag in the halls. We knew that this was our last full family gathering in the city where we all grew up. It made us weepy. I felt another heaviness. Judi and I would not have twin time any more. What would we have to talk about now that the Parent Project was over? Everyone else milled around but I stuck close to Judi and held her hand.

The Catholic Mass the next day featured a string of priests lined up before the altar, with my brother the priest in charge. John, the light of her life. Family filled the front rows. Then we all went in a line of cars with our lights on to the cemetery plot. Judi and I had chosen it together, the year before. We liked it because it looked over Calgary and was close to the huge white cross where a special Mass was said by the bishop every year on All Souls Day. With binoculars, Judi could see it from her bedroom window. Matt placed the little box of ashes into the hole chipped out of the frozen ground, and quipped, "There, she's planted."

Matt snapped the band of tension that had bound my heart and I let myself do what I had not done in a while. I laughed.

Back at the hotel where the beer now lay in tepid water and pizza crusts littered the carpet, we munched on leftovers from the funeral lunch. Picking at the remains of a sandwich tray, Matt mused, "What about that crazy wind that gusted just when I put Mom in the hole? Did anyone else notice that?" I said I felt it, too. "Did it come from the Maritimes, do you think?" Ears around the room pricked up as Matt and I began to talk about east winds in Calgary, agreeing that it was as weird as it was cold. "Maybe it's a sign," Matt suggested.

John was impatient with us. Winds blew. We should not start making up stories. Matt said he preferred talking about the weather than sitting around moping. "What kind party poopers are you guys?" he added. Chris said he hadn't felt anything special. It was just a lousy January afternoon on the top of a Calgary hill. Nancy wanted this discussion about signs to be recorded on tape, for a project someday maybe. My husband Ed fiddled with his camera but said there was not enough light in the room. Steve fiddled with his cellphone. "Eastwind would make a good password," he mused. "Strong."

I cleared my throat, wondering if I should say what was on my mind. "Why not?" I told myself, "It's your truth, speak!" So, still hesitating, I began. "Mom had a favourite caregiver named Cheryl. She had a tattoo on her arm that she said was about the four directions. East is a big-deal direction, well, they all have meaning." I explained how east was the direction of light in her indigenous culture, and west was the direction of wisdom. "East heading west," I paused. "I'm just saying..." Chris shrugged and looked at his watch, "Time to move on," he said, promising to keep in touch and pulling on his boots. "This party is over." Soon we had all hugged and gone our separate ways.

I don't know if that east wind was a last message as Mom's spirit flew or if it was just a quirk of the weather that day. I do know that with that gust, our Parent Project was over. Both Mom and Dad had completed their journeys, and so had my twin and me. We had all learned about love and caregiving at the edge of life. There was something else I knew for sure. I would never be quite the same.

Praise for *The Dwindling*

Gail Sheehy, author of *Passages*, and *The Caregiving Passage*.

A daring yet compassionate memoir for everyone called to make the caregiving passage with a slow-dying parent. Dunnett will lead you through the isolation to find quality care and tender connections. And keep you company!

Stephen Kiernan, author of *Last Rights* and *The Baker's Secret*.

Some books are like mirrors: as we read their pages we see ourselves. For people everywhere with aging parents, The Dwindling is just such a book, reflecting one family's fervent, earnest, and taxing struggle to care for a mother and father as their days begin to dwindle. Between the habits of clinicians and the complexity of health care financing, its a frustrating job that requires a deep reservoir of love and self-sacrifice. But this book shows a way to find the strength and patience. For those not lucky enough to have Janet Dunnett by their side, her book will serve as a useful ally just when their loved ones need one most.

Eric Wasylenko, MD, Clinical Assistant Professor,
Division of Palliative Medicine, Department of Oncology,
Cumming School of Medicine, University of Calgary.

*This book is a must-read about personal revelation, the
healing and completion of relationships, and the attitude of
loving service required to 'walk with' frail parents on their
relentless path towards death.*

*The discovered strength and wisdom, acknowledgement of
failures and celebration of 'sisterhood' reveals the growth
that occurs in all of us – at all stages of life. What shines
through is the need to always question and push the formal
health care system in a search for quality and safety, during
what increasingly will be a partnership of care amongst
families, communities and professionals. The honesty and
wry humour with which Ms. Dunnett shares her family's
story will assist all readers to pack some extra doses of
courage, and some practical advice, for their own companionship journey.*

John Sloan, MD, Physician and Author of *A Bitter Pill. How the
Medical System is Failing the Elderly.* Find him at www.sunshiners.ca

*Janet Dunnett has written a captivating and honest account
of caring for her frail and dying parents. I know from recent
personal experience that this is a monstrously difficult thing
to do, even for a doctor trained in geriatrics. I have to learn
everything about frailty all over again in doing it for my
own in-laws. How much more of an uphill battle it is for*

everyone else is described with sympathetic humour and love in this important book. Required reading if you are, or are going to be, looking after elderly loved ones. To save the healthcare system and return dignity and kindness to the end of life we need more books like it, and more courageous people like Ms. Dunnett in the world.

Joanne Lynn, MD, MA, MS. Director of the Centre for Elder Care and Advanced Illness in the Altarum Institute, Washington, D.C. Find her at www.medicaring.org

We need to tell stories, to get people familiar with the language and the experiences of end of life, and the evaluation of the merits of current care pathways. This book is just such a story.

Christine Osborne RN, Gerontology specialist and boomer caregiver.

My sisters and I faced many of the same challenges "Goliath" presented to the author. Our mother too required increasing care for her complex needs as she began to fail. We, too, tried to look after her at home, but that lasted only days. Janet Dunnett's description of sleeping on the floor in her mother's room, in case she should need her in the night, took me right back to the few nights I spent in a similar situation at my sister's house, where we had installed a hospital bed, a wheeled commode and transfer belts. It's amazing to me that the author was able to keep it up for so long.

I really hope this book makes it onto mainstream book-shelves, as I think there is so much we can all learn from and share, especially as we face our own dwindling.

Beth Diamond, President National Diamond Associates, Calgary.

"The Dwindling" is lyrical, vivid and moving. Though personal, this story has a universal tone and truth that I believe will make it relevant to all readers. In Dunnett's hands, slow decline becomes a fast-paced, funny, moving and engaging narrative with rich characters that gripped me from the get-go. Past and present was woven into a tapestry of back and forth. I couldn't put it down!

This is not an ordinary book. On the surface, it will certainly inspire and help those who read it. Just as important, it will move, entertain and engage all readers facing not just this circumstance but any challenge involving complex relationships.

Thank you for writing it.